# Understanding Pain

American Academy of Neurology Press (AAN)
Quality of Life Guides

Lisa M. Shulman, MD
*Series Editor*

ALZHEIMER'S DISEASE
Paul Dash, MD and Nicole Villemarette-Pittman, PhD

AMYOTROPHIC LATERAL SCLEROSIS
Robert G. Miller, MD, Deborah Gelinas, MD,
and Patricia O'Connor, RN

EPILEPSY
Ilo E. Leppik, MD

GUILLAIN-BARRÉ SYNDROME
Gareth John Parry, MB, ChB, FRACP and Joel S. Steinberg, MD, PhD

MIGRAINE AND OTHER HEADACHES
William B. Young, MD and Stephen D. Silberstein, MD

PERIPHERAL NEUROPATHY
Norman Latov, MD, PhD

RESTLESS LEGS SYNDROME
Mark J. Buchfuhrer, MD, Wayne A. Henning, MD, PhD,
and Clete A. Kushida, MD

STROKE
Louis R. Caplan, MD

# Understanding Pain

## *What It Is, Why It Happens, and How It's Managed*

### HARRY J. GOULD III, MD, PhD

Associate Professor of Neurology
Director
LSU Pain Mastery Center
Louisiana State University Health Sciences Center
New Orleans, Louisiana


### LISA M. SHULMAN, MD
Series Editor

Associate Professor of Neurology
Rosalyn Newman Distinguished Scholar in Parkinson's Disease
Co-Director, Maryland Parkinson's Disease
and Movement Disorders Center
The University of Maryland Medical Center
Baltimore, Maryland

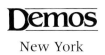

New York

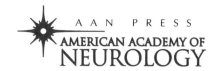

AAN PRESS
AMERICAN ACADEMY OF
NEUROLOGY

**Library of Congress Cataloging-in-Publication Data**

Gould, Harry J.
  Understanding pain : what it is, why it happens, and how it's managed / Harry J. Gould, III.
      p. cm.
  Includes bibliographical references.
  ISBN-13: 978-1-932603-58-3 (pbk. : alk. paper)
  ISBN-10: 1-932603-58-1 (pbk. : alk. paper)
  1. Pain—Popular works. 2. Pain—Treatment—Popular works. I. Title.
  RB127.G68 2007
  616'.0472—dc22

                                                              2006033199

Special discounts on bulk quantities of Demos Medical Publishing books are available to corporations, professional associations, pharmaceutical companies, health care organizations, and other qualifying groups. For details, please contact:

Special Sales Department
Demos Medical Publishing
386 Park Avenue South, Suite 301
New York, NY 10016
Phone: 800-532-8663, 212-683-0072
Fax: 212-683-0118
Email: orderdept@demosmedpub.com

Made in the United States of America
06 07 08 09 10    5 4 3 2 1

To Trevor and Laura

# Contents

Contents

# About the AAN Press Quality of Life Guides

## IN THE SPIRIT OF THE DOCTOR-PATIENT PARTNERSHIP

THE BETTER-INFORMED PATIENT is often able to play a vital role in his or her own care. This is especially the case with neurologic disorders, for which effective management of disease can be promoted—indeed, *enhanced*—through patient education and involvement.

In the spirit of the partnership-in-care between physicians and patients, the American Academy of Neurology Press is pleased to produce a series of "Quality of Life" guides on an array of diseases and ailments that affect the brain and central nervous system. The series, produced in partnership with Demos Medical Publishing, answers a number of basic and important questions faced by patients and their families.

Additionally, the authors, most of whom are physicians and all of whom are experts in the areas in which they write, provide a detailed discussion of the disorder, its causes, and the course it may follow. You also find strategies for coping with the disorder and handling a number of nonmedical issues.

The result: As a reader, you will be able to develop a framework for understanding the disease and become better prepared to manage the life changes associated with it.

## ABOUT THE AMERICAN ACADEMY OF NEUROLOGY (AAN)

The American Academy of Neurology is the premier organization for neurologists worldwide. In addition to support of educational and scientific advances, the AAN—along with its sister organization, the AAN Foundation—is a strong advocate of public education and a leading supporter of research for breakthroughs in neurologic patient care.

More information on the activities of the AAN is available on our website, www.aan.com. For a better understanding of common disorders of the brain, as well as to learn about people living with these disorders, please turn to the AAN Foundation's website, www.thebrainmatters.org.

## ABOUT NEUROLOGY AND NEUROLOGISTS

Neurology is the medical specialty associated with disorders of the brain and central nervous system. Neurologists are medical doctors with specialized training in the diagnosis, treatment, and management of patients suffering from neurologic disease.

Lisa M. Shulman, M.D.
*Series Editor*
*AAN Press Quality of Life Guides*

# Preface

*May not cure the malady or find reason for the pain, but dare to share a moment
to understand the strain. If only for a moment, perhaps for just a day, might
hold a hand and free a smile, lift a spirit worn by pain.*

—*HJB III*

IN RECENT YEARS, there has been a growing interest in the subject of
pain from several perspectives. There is greater public awareness that
pain is an important clinical and social problem. People have become
aware that pain is frequently under-recognized, under-treated, and all
too often either ignored or managed only passively in relation to treating other primary medical conditions. As a result, uncontrolled pain has
placed an overwhelming psychological and economic burden on society
in the form of increasing healthcare cost and loss of productivity. There
is also a growing awareness of the need and an increased expectation for
better pain management along with the recognition that resources are
currently available to improve pain control and a patient's quality of life
if such resources are not withheld from management plans. Indeed,
there is a growing opinion that individuals have a right to adequate pain
management, yet there is a general lack of knowledge about the complex nature of pain and how it should be managed.

The increased focus on pain and pain management within the community at large has led to several important avenues of investigation.
First, there has been an upsurge in basic research efforts with a goal to
improve our understanding of how a noxious stimulus is received and
processed by the nervous system, integrated with past experience, and
then uniquely perceived by an individual.

In this context, much research has focused on how and why it is that
some painful conditions are transient and thereby protective and beneficial, whereas other conditions set the stage for the development of pain

states that are chronic and destructive to the quality of life for the sufferer as well as to related families and society as a whole. Second, as a result of basic research efforts, the pharmacological armamentarium used to treat pain has expanded greatly. Many pharmacological agents that had never been considered as pain relievers have been found to have analgesic properties and as such, have contributed significantly to improved pain control. The observation that the mechanisms through which drugs produce their primary effect, also produce an analgesic effect by influencing the processing of a painful stimulus, has led to changes in our approach to the clinical assessment of pain. This change in the approach to pain assessment challenges both the patient and the healthcare professional, to be more cognizant of the variable and complex nature of a perceived painful condition in order to communicate more effectively and thereby improve the management of pain for the betterment of all. The correlation of clinical responses to treatment protocols, in light of new understanding about the basic mechanisms that underlie the development and management of pain, has been the impetus for increased efforts in drug discovery and the development of alternative management protocols, both pharmacological and non-pharmacological, for improved patient care. Third, the increased focus on providing adequate pain control to greater numbers of individuals has led to a greater need for the education of clinicians, patients, and society as a whole about the beneficial and the potentially negative effects of providing adequate analgesic medication.

This book has been written to provide a source to the general public for developing an understanding of the scope of what it is that we are treating when we say we are treating pain. Details about the anatomy and physiology of the pain pathways will be presented to help explain where medications might act upon the pain pathways to produce an analgesic effect, and why they would be considered for the treatment of pain. This book is not designed to be an exhaustive source for the researcher or clinician, but instead, one in which patients, their families, and friends may obtain information to aid in developing an understanding that will lead to a more informed and active role in the management of pain. Healthcare providers may also find the information presented relevant to issues of pain management as it pertains to their practice. I hope that the information provided in this book will help establish a common foundation for dialogue between patients and healthcare providers. For example, what are the important features about pain that should be recognized, communicated, and discussed, between patient and healthcare provider? What options are available in the management of pain of different types? Why are certain treatment options, pharmacological and non-pharmacological, considered in the management of pain? The book will also attempt to dispel some of the myths about the use of analgesic medications, present their appropriate use and potential benefits when used in the treatment of prolonged, uncontrolled pain.

Harry J. Gould III, MD, PhD

# Acknowledgments

I WOULD LIKE TO THANK my wife Anne, Henry E. "Hammerin' Hank" Miller, Jr., Dennis Paul, Jane Sumner, and Shantel Watson for their time, effort, and encouragement, and their helpful comments and suggestions in the preparation of the manuscript and Eugene New for his advise and talent in the preparation of the illustrations. I thank Austin J. Sumner for his continued support and for the opportunity to attempt this project. Finally, I want to recognize and thank those who over the years have entrusted their care to me. I thank them for allowing me the privilege to learn from them while attempting to help, although all too often not as successfully as hoped, to reduce the burden of their pain, if only for a few moments in time. They have taught me much more than many books such as this one, have been important inspirations in the writing of this book, and without whom this project would not have been possible.

# CHAPTER 1

# Pain Defined—What Are We Treating?

Pain is a complex sensory and emotional experience that is essential for survival. Although unpleasant, pain is the sense that tells us when we have already or are in the process of injuring ourselves. It warns us that something must be done to prevent further injury or compels us to seek treatment for the condition responsible for the pain. Despite the significance of pain as a factor in human survival, only recently has it received attention as a major contributor to the cost of health care and a clinical entity worthy of specific attention.

Virtually everyone has experienced pain at some time in his life, yet despite each person's experience, very few people are aware of pain's multifaceted nature. This lack of understanding frequently leads to inadequate treatment, inadequate pain relief, and frustration on the part of both sufferer and health care provider.

It is important to realize that pain perception is influenced by culture, situation, and past experience; thus, it is uniquely experienced by each individual. As in viewing a work of art or listening to a composition of music, the experience is perceived differently by different individuals—and possibly differently when experienced by the same individual at different times. Unfortunately, those suffering pain often are unable to effectively describe the hurt they feel in a way that conveys the essence of their experience to someone else, who listens from the perspective of a different life experience. The problem of communication is not, however, solely the fault of the person experiencing pain. It is shared as well by health care professionals who receive limited training in how to properly assess pain and manage it effectively. As a result, health care providers typically do not pursue the lines of questioning

1

necessary to draw out important information about the patient's pain, other than to determine its intensity. This leads to a situation in which every pain is treated similarly using various painkillers.

Much of the difficulty in providing adequate pain management lies in the fact that it was not until 1979 that the International Association for the Study of Pain arrived at a comprehensive definition of pain that encompasses the complexity of the experience. Pain thus defined is "a sensory and emotional experience that is associated with actual or potential tissue injury and is described in such terms" (International Association for the Study of Pain. *Pain* 6:249, 1979). Implicit in the definition is that, although tissue injury most often is associated intimately with the perception of pain, it is not essential to the experience. In addition, the emotional state of an individual plays an important role in pain perception. For example, numerous instances occur when pain is present in the absence of a noxious stimulus (a stimulus sufficient to cause an uncomfortable sensation and potentially damage tissue), such as the heartache at the loss of a loved one or the physical discomfort that many experience prior to a stressful event. Conversely, at times a noxious stimulus is present, yet no pain is perceived. It might seem surprising, but it is not uncommon for individuals who suffer significant trauma, such as a gun shot wound, to experience no pain until some time after the actual injury. Therefore, *pain is what the sufferer says it is*—and the evaluation and management of the problem should start with this.

## CLASSIFICATIONS OR TYPES OF PAIN

Pain is not always what it seems, and it can be classified in many different ways. Each classification, although frequently overlapping another, provides a unique hint about what is responsible for the pain and how it may be treated best.

## Pain Can Be Defined with Respect to Time

At a basic level, pain can be described in the context of how long it has been present. *Acute pain* occurs at the time of an injury and lasts for only that period of time during which the reason for the pain is present. Stubbing a toe, cutting a finger, or receiving a burn result in forms of acute pain. Acute pain can occur as an isolated, one-time event, or it may reoccur as a series time-limited events that manifest in a similar or *stereotypic* fashion at varying intervals.

*Recurrent acute pain* can occur regularly, as in the case of monthly menstrual pains, or it can reoccur irregularly, as in the case of chest pain related to episodes of insufficient blood supply to the heart muscle (angina) or migraine headaches.

In contrast, *persistent* or *chronic pain* occurs for prolonged periods of time. The duration of the pain necessary for a diagnosis of chronic pain varies. Although the diagnosis of chronic pain classically has been reserved for pain that persists for more than 3 to 6 months under any condition, current thinking suggests that pain should be considered chronic when it arises from an isolated injury (e.g., trauma-induced pain, such as a fracture or sprain) and lasts longer than what would be predicted for recovery from the initial injury. The chronic pain associated with a permanent or progressive condition (e.g., cancer or arthritis) and therefore constantly present becomes, by virtue of its unrelenting nature, a disease entity worthy of treatment in its own right.

It is important to realize that acute pain may be experienced and coexist with chronic pain, and that the conditions are not mutually exclusive. Indeed, the occurrence of an acute increase in pain in someone suffering from a life-long disease is often an indication of an alteration in the course of the underlying disease process and is worthy of reassessment.

## Pain Can Be Defined with Respect to the Portion of the Body Involved

Pain also may be described in relationship to its distribution in the body. Pain located in a restricted region, such as the head, chest, back, or limb, is described as *focal pain*. The distribution of the pain can be precisely localized, as with cuts, scrapes, and fractures, or it can be distributed more broadly, as in the typical presentation of a "stomach-ache." Focal pain may be felt in a single location, or it may be perceived at more than one site. In these cases, the pain is described as *multifocal*.

Pain is not always confined to a particular region, but may shift from one primary site to involve another. Pain that spreads from an initial focus is said to *radiate* or extend from the focus of origin. Patterns of extension can be helpful in determining the source of the pain. Some pain radiates from the borders of the primary focus to varying degrees depending on body position or activity, whereas other pain radiates within the distribution of particular nerves or nerve roots. The latter type of pain is characteristic of a nerve injury. This pain usually has a sudden onset and, when it occurs, lasts for only short periods. Most people have experienced this type of pain when they experience trauma to the inner aspect of the elbow or "hit their funny bone." The sensation results from trauma to the ulnar nerve at the elbow; it produces an uncomfortable sensation both at the point of impact and down the forearm into the fourth and fifth fingers of the hand. If similar trauma involves a primary nerve root close to the spinal column, as can occur in association with a herniated intervertebral disk ("slipped disk"), the affected area of radiation is that of the entire nerve root. The pain of sciatica is perhaps the best recognized example of this type of pain. In sciatica, general, persistent discomfort in the low back is accompanied by shock-like sensations of varying frequencies that shoot down the leg and into the toes.

Similar radiating pain also can occur following injury to the central nervous system (CNS) following a stroke or mechanical trauma to the spinal cord or brain. The resulting pattern of pain involves those portions of the body that are served by the affected neuronal pathways. This typically involves all body regions below the site of injury on the side related to the injured pathways. Pain of this nature is said to have a *central pattern of distribution*, because it reflects the characteristic distribution of those CNS pathways involved, rather than a pattern of the individual nerves that supply skin, muscles, and bones.

Pain resulting from a focal injury also may be felt at a location distant from the site of tissue injury. In other words, tissue injury at one site can produce pain in a region separate and distinct from that involved in the injury. This type of pain is called *referred pain.* The patterns of referral, if recognized, can be important in determining the underlying cause of the pain. Perhaps the best known example of referred pain is that associated with tissue injury resulting from insufficient blood supply to heart muscle during a heart attack. Heart pain is perceived not only in the chest, but frequently in the arm and jaw as well. A less well-known example of referred pattern is that of pain perceived in the scapula or shoulder blade associated with injury to the tissues of the gall bladder.

## Pain Can Be Described with Respect to the Tissue Type Involved

*Somatic pain* is pain associated with structures of the body wall. It is usually precisely localized by the individual, felt close to the time of injury, and of relatively high intensity. The rapid and precisely localizing feature of this pain is important because the outer body structures—the somatic parts—provide the first line of defense for the individual against injury. Because they are used to explore the environment and are thus more likely to be injured, somatic parts (such as the limbs) are endowed with an extensive nerve supply to monitor for potential injury. Because of the greater nerve supply, information conveyed to the brain from somatic parts is very complete; all stimulation, both painful and nonpainful, is felt readily. The information transmitted along the nerves allows for precise localization and assessment of the type of stimulus producing an injury. In contrast, when similar stimulation is presented to internal or visceral organs such as blood vessels, liver, spleen, and intestines, which have many fewer nerves relegated to monitoring their condition, the resulting *visceral pain* is usually perceived as vague and poorly localized. The idea that internal organs are monitored by fewer nerves is reinforced by the fact that non-noxious stimulation of visceral structures, like the transit of food through the intestinal system, is seldom perceived at a conscious level. Only when non-noxious stimuli are presented at the entrance and exit regions of the digestive system, close to the body surface (the somatic portion of the digestive system), are they consciously perceived.

## Pain Can Be Described by the Way It Is Generated

Pain associated with actual or potential tissue injury in the presence of a normally functioning nervous system is called *nociceptive pain* (from the

Latin *noci* meaning to injure and *capere* meaning to receive). Everyone is familiar with nociceptive pain. In its acute form, this type of pain enables one to avoid injury or to minimize the injury resulting from potentially destructive forces. This type of pain, unless associated with a progressive process such as arthritis or cancer, is usually worst when it starts and resolves after the wound has healed. A good example of this type of pain is the pain associated with the fracture of a bone. Immediate and exquisitely intense pain occurs at the time of injury, but the pain decreases as healing progresses until such time as the bone has healed and pain is no longer perceived. This type of pain can be effectively managed with typical painkillers.

Pain also can be produced in the absence of ongoing tissue injury when the nerves that usually convey pain signals from a site of injury are spontaneously activated. Because the signal is related to the functional disturbance of nerves, this type of pain is called *neuropathic pain*. It can occur as a result of an injury to either the brain and spinal cord or to the peripheral nerves, and it results in spontaneous activity within the pain pathways. The abnormal activity of the nervous system may be, and frequently is, present in the absence of any ongoing tissue injury. Spontaneous neuronal activity—and consequently pain of neuropathic origin—is much less responsive to typical painkillers. If neuropathic pain is untreated, the spontaneous activity can sensitize other nerves that transmit pain signals. In those cases, noxious stimuli are perceived more intensely than would otherwise be predicted or at levels of intensity that should not be uncomfortable. The perception of a nonpainful stimulus as painful is a phenomenon called *allodynia*. Unfortunately, because objective evidence to substantiate an individual's complaint of neuropathic pain is frequently lacking, and the response to standard pain medicines is unsatisfactory, these individuals often are viewed as either having fabricated the complaint or to be suffering from a psychological problem. Treatment for these individuals often is refused or inadequate. If ineffectively or inadequately managed, neuropathic pain may become worse and may become permanent.

Individuals with psychological conditions such as anxiety and depression frequently report experiencing pain in various regions of the body. This is called *psychogenic pain*. It is therefore important to consider a psychological basis for the pain complaint when objective evidence is absent to support the presence of nociceptive pain, the symptomatology is inconsistent with neuropathic pain, and there occurs a lack of response to treatment that would be predicted to produce reasonable relief from the pain. The descriptions of symptoms related to psychogenic pain infrequently conform to known patterns of nerve distribution and have characteristics atypical of either nociceptive or neuropathic pain. The fact that pain is of psychogenic origin, however, does not imply that the pain does not exist, nor does it mean that the pain is less uncomfortable to the one perceiving it. It is important to acknowledge that psychogenic pain, if left untreated, is just as destructive to the individual's quality of life as pain arising from a clearly defined origin. A concerted effort to find the condition that underlies the pain is essential and justified.

Finally, some pain complaints defy the diagnostic skills of the health care provider and cannot be characterized as nociceptive, neuropathic, or psychogenic in origin. It is likely that such conditions defy classification because, at this time, either our level of understanding of the pain processing system is insufficient to determine an underlying cause or our technology has not yet developed to a level that enables us to further classify the pain. This pain is referred to as *idiopathic pain* (from the Greek *idio* meaning own or peculiar and *pathos* meaning disease or functional disturbance). Although the basis for the pain cannot be determined, it is nonetheless important to manage. *Pain is what the patient says it is* until such time as it is determined that the pain complaint has been knowingly fabricated for secondary gain (that is, made up for purposes of achieving personal reward or satisfaction). Then it is considered *factitious pain* or *malingering*.

The role of the health care provider in managing pain is to believe the patient and to diagnose the pain in the best way possible. The role of the patient in managing pain is to be a careful observer and reporter of the pain being experienced. With good communication, the most effective treatment plan is likely to be determined and the best outcome realized.

7

CHAPTER 2

# The Evaluation— What Should I Tell My Doctor?

Less than 30 years has passed since a comprehensive definition of pain has been established. Therefore, it is not surprising that few people who experience pain are aware of what is important to convey to their health care provider when seeking assistance for relief of pain. Irrespective of the definition, the reporting of pain is frequently minimized for several reasons; this lessens the likelihood of successful pain control. First, in many situations and in many societies, an admission of pain is viewed as a form of personal weakness; therefore, it either is not admitted, not reported, or both. Second, many individuals who suffer pain, fear, not unreasonably, that something serious and perhaps life-threatening is causing the pain; by complaining about the pain, the attention of the health care provider will be diverted from adequate treatment of the source of the problem. Third, many individuals fear taking medications for pain. They may have observed complications of medications, or remember when medications were given to dying family members; thus, they associate the administration of strong painkillers with adverse effects and end of life. They also may have heard or seen reports of people who "get hooked" on pain medications. Fourth, people generally like to be viewed as "good patients," and they may believe that they will not be viewed as such if they always seem to complain about pain. Finally, most people learn to explain or express their pain through the observations of how others, such as parents, caregivers, and acquaintances, describe theirs. It is essential, therefore, to realize that because pain is complex in nature, it is important to provide as much information as possible if the goal is to achieve the best relief possible.

*What information is important to convey when seeking help for pain relief, and how might this information be collected and organized for presentation to a health care provider?* Once an initial pain problem is recognized and medical assistance is deemed necessary, it is a good idea to begin keeping a daily record of the pain. Because pain that is no longer being experienced is usually only vaguely remembered, and therefore difficult to recall, it is helpful to keep notes about the pain experience during the time that it is being experienced. This record should be maintained until the pain is evaluated for the first time and throughout treatment. In general, an assessment once a day for a 24-hour period is sufficient to provide information about the progress of the pain—whether it is improving, worsening, or fluctuating from its start to the time of first evaluation. It is helpful to know the highest level, the lowest level, and the average level of pain (the level experienced for most of the day) over the course of each 24-hour period. Time spent in this activity should not take more than a few minutes each day. The descriptions of the pain should not be edited after writing. It is important to avoid dwelling on and thereby enhancing the pain problem. This baseline information provides a clue to the underlying cause of the pain and a point of reference upon which changes in response to treatment can be compared.

## IMPORTANT COMPONENTS OF THE PAIN EXPERIENCE

### The Intensity of the Pain

For the one suffering the pain, the most important aspect to report is its intensity. This is the "how much" of pain; how badly it hurts. No objective ways to measure pain intensity exist, since any individual's physiological and emotional response, even to a particular measured painful stimulus such as a calibrated heat source or mechanical stimulator, can vary with time, situation, and presentation. Assessments of pain intensity are therefore subjective and based on the individual's past experience and internal standard. Several methods frequently used to assist in

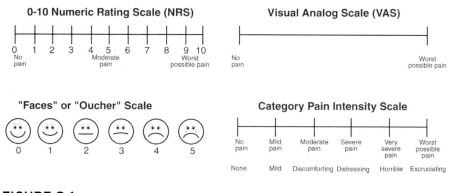

## FIGURE 2-1

Pain Assessment Scales. (Modified from National Initiative on Pain Control™. Used with the permission of Thomson Postgraduate Services®).

the attempt to communicate the level of intensity perceived by one individual to another are illustrated in Figure 2-1. The choice of one method over another frequently is based on its ease of use both for the health care provider and for the pain sufferer.

The most frequently used method is the *numeric rating scale (NRS)*. This method assumes a range between 0 and 10, in which 0 represents no pain and 10 represents the worst pain imagined. The individual assigns a number along that continuum to correspond to the pain level experienced. In general, levels of 1 to 3 are used to report pain in the mild range, 4 to 6 describes moderate pain, and 7 to 10 denotes severe pain.

Another method of measurement is the *visual analogue scale (VAS)*. For this, a line, typically 10 centimeters long, is drawn on a piece of paper. One end of the line is designated "No Pain" and the other "Worst Pain." The individual then marks a point on the line that corresponds to the level of perceived pain. The distance between the "No Pain" end of the line and the mark is recorded as the pain intensity score.

The third method in frequent use is the *faces of pain* or *"oucher" scale*. This method is very useful for those who have difficulty conceptualizing numbers or are unable to understand the other scales due to a lack of development, education, or varying states of dementia. This scale is used most frequently with children. It presents a series of cartoon faces that depict a smiling face at the "No Pain" end and a face that is crying at the

"Worst Pain" end. The patient selects the face that depicts the expression that corresponds with his level of pain.

Finally, a *category scale* provides another way to attempt to measure pain intensity. For this method, a series of words frequently used to describe pain of different levels—mild, discomforting, distressing, horrible, and excruciating—is provided. The individual selects and records the most appropriate word to describe his pain.

Other methods that expand upon these concepts are available and may be useful for selected individuals, but are beyond the scope of this book. Two basic principles may serve as a guide in measuring pain intensity. First, the method that is easiest to use and is the simplest to understand is most likely to be used by the pain sufferer, and therefore is the most likely method to provide reliable information. Second, the use of more than one method increases the consistency or reliability of the observation.

## The Quality of the Pain

Perhaps the most important characteristic of the pain to identify and report for the health care provider is its quality. This is the "what it feels like" of pain; what is the sensation? Typically, patients say that their pain is a hurt; a big hurt, an annoying hurt, a terrible hurt, which is an expression of discomfort and intensity. This is of little help in determining a possible cause and potential treatment for the pain. In general, all pain hurts, but different injuries produce different kinds of hurt. For example, the quality of a hurt felt when one places a hand on a hot stove is different from the quality of hurt related to a knife cut or an electric shock. The quality of the sensation indicates the nature of an injury to the health care provider evaluating the pain. The pain patient must provide "the eyes" that the health care provider will use to determine the source of the pain. Many words are used to describe the quality of pain, such as burning, crushing, stabbing, twisting, and aching. Indeed, over 200 words have been used to describe the quality of the pain experience. The McGill Pain Questionnaire has organized these descriptors into 20 different groups—for example, Group 2: jumping, flashing, shooting; Group 19: cool, cold, freezing—in an effort to elicit information that will help diagnose and manage pain. A concerted effort to identify as many character-istics of the painful sensation as possible will go a long way toward estab-lishing a diagnosis and improving the likelihood of relief.

## The Location and Distribution of the Pain

This is the "where does it hurt" of pain; how much of the body is involved? Whenever possible, it is helpful to define those portions of the body involved with pain. This is most easily accomplished by drawing an outline on an illustration of the body surface that defines the boundaries of the painful region or regions. As illustrated in Figure 2-2, the regions

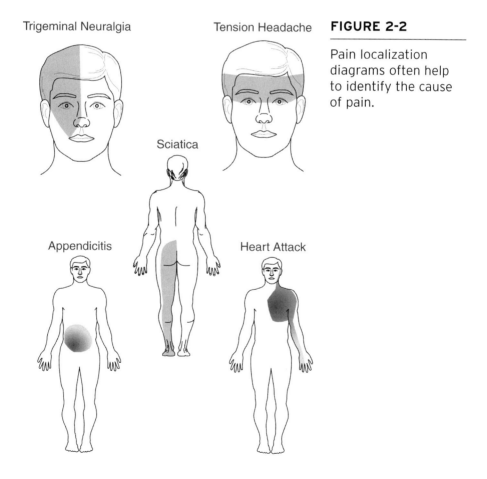

Trigeminal Neuralgia

Tension Headache

Sciatica

Appendicitis

Heart Attack

**FIGURE 2-2**

Pain localization diagrams often help to identify the cause of pain.

thus defined often provide clues to the underlying cause of the pain. For instance, "deep, stabbing" pain that involves the low back and "shoots down" the posterior or back of the leg is characteristic of pain associated with a herniated disk between the lowest lumbar vertebra and the sacrum. In contrast, a "vise-like pressure" pain that wraps around the head like a hat-band frequently is reported by individuals suffering tension-type headaches. The patterns provided by the pain sufferer frequently guide the health care provider to ask more specific questions about past medical history, occupation, activities, lifestyle, stressors, and previous trauma. This line of questioning is likely to indicate further testing to elucidate the cause of the pain.

## The Duration, Frequency, and Pattern of the Pain

This is the "how long has it been there" of pain. Three factors are important when describing pain from this perspective. The first factor is related to each individual pain episode. It is important to define the time course of each painful event—when it starts, how long it usually lasts, and what happens during the episode, as illustrated in Figure 2-3 for a migraine headache. Acute pain may come on quickly and last seconds to minutes, or it may build gradually in intensity over minutes to hours to days.

The second factor is related to the pattern in which the pain episodes occur. Recurring pain may come at regular intervals, as in the case of menstrual cramps or headaches that are related to seasonal allergies or to the time of day (see Fig. 2-3). Recurrent pain also may occur irregularly and unpredictably, as in many cases of migraine headache and muscle spasm. It is important to identify the general pattern of pain that occurs in each episode and between episodes, because changes in such patterns may indicate a change in the course of the disease or that a new condition is emerging. Acute, short-lived, infrequent pain episodes generally should be treated early when they occur and during the time they are present.

Chronic pain should be described similarly to acute pain with respect to time—when it started, how long it has been present, and what has happened since it began—but with the understanding that fundamental differences exist between acute and chronic pain conditions. With

14

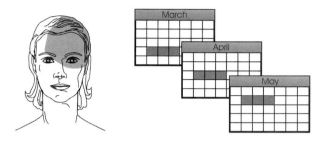

## FIGURE 2-3

Summary of the distribution, duration (12 hours), frequency (3 days/month), and pattern (every fourth week) of a migraine headache related to the menstrual cycle.

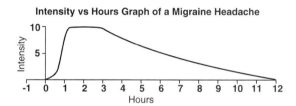

chronic pain, at least a portion of the pain problem is always present. In addition, and in virtually all cases, superimposed upon the persistent pain are episodes in which pain similar to the background pain increases in intensity, then later returns to its baseline level. Periods also may occur during which a pain of a different quality occurs in addition to the constant pain sensation. The timing of the fluctuations in pain intensity and quality within a pattern of chronic pain—the frequency of exacerbations and the times of the day when they occur—is important to identify. Variations in the pattern of pain in response to treatment is a good indicator of whether benefit is being achieved or perhaps which portion of the treatment is most likely to be providing the greatest benefit. Frequent acute pain episodes and persistent chronic pain conditions should be managed very similarly from a perspective of prophylaxis or prevention, because it is important to reduce the frequency and intensity of exacerbations and to achieve the lowest levels of persistent pain.

Regardless of the type of pain problem, the third factor—the overall duration of the problem and how it has changed with time—provides clues to the pathology that may be responsible for the pain. Furthermore, the duration of the problem serves as an indicator of prognosis for recovery, progress of the underlying disease, and the potential for a response to treatment. For example, pain of sudden onset that persists for months to years may well be related to trauma from a fall, a lifting injury, or a motor vehicle accident. Conversely, pain that has a vague point of onset and builds gradually with time is more frequently associated with an underlying medical condition or disease process, such as cancer or arthritis. Conditions that worsen rapidly are likely to become debilitating earlier than are conditions that appear to remain stable for months to years. Conditions that have persisted for longer than 6 months are less likely to resolve or respond effectively to treatment than are those that show immediate improvement with early treatment.

## What Has Been Tried to Relieve the Pain?

Unless an obvious cause for the pain being experienced requires urgent medical attention, as in the case of a fractured bone, most individuals prefer not to involve a physician without first attempting to treat the problem themselves. Home remedies and over-the-counter medications often are tried with varying degrees of success. During the self-treating process, one can usually identify those things that have made the problem worse, have made the problem better, or seemed to have had no effect. For example, if certain positions or treatments have exacerbated the pain, obviously, these treatment options should be avoided where possible. To the statement, "Doc, when I do this, the pain gets worse," one might well answer, "Don't do that." Not all problems can be managed that easily, but avoiding known exacerbating behavior when possible may aid in healing and reduce the pain to more manageable levels. For those who have had previous evaluations and treatments, it is useful to know what already has been tried to alleviate the pain, especially if the problem has been recurrent or chronic. A list should be compiled that summarizes past treatments, including previous medications, physical and occupational therapy, psychological management and biofeedback, injections (of what drug and where it was injected), surgical procedures, and alternative therapies such as acupuncture or hypnosis, and an indication of whether the treatment helped, hurt, or had no effect.

If the treatment helped, how much did it help and for how long was benefit noted? For example, "When I use two tablets of ibuprofen, my pain usually decreases by approximately two pain levels, from a 3 to a 1, for about 2 hours." or "My pain resolved completely for about 1 week after Dr. Jones gave me a steroid injection in my shoulder." Certain treatments may provide only partial improvement, but their benefit may be enhanced if treatments are combined. It is, therefore, helpful to know if past treatments were implemented separately and sequentially or in combination.

If no benefit was noticed, the characteristics of the treatment should be identified—how frequently was the method tried and for how long. For example, "I participated in physical therapy three times a week for 4 months and did not notice any improvement." In the case of medications, it is important to identify:

- The medication used
- The highest dose of the medication tried
- The length of the treatment period of each medication
- Whether the medications were used one at a time or in combination with other medications
- Why the treatment was discontinued (e.g., adverse effects or lack of benefit)

Individuals often are prescribed appropriate medications for the treatment of their pain, but in the absence of adverse effects, the treatment may be abandoned prior to reaching a dose necessary to achieve pain relief. In these situations, some of the previously ineffective medications may be retried at more appropriate doses with the likelihood of success. Alternatively, inappropriate medication trials for a particular type of pain occasionally have been attempted, predictably without success. An expected lack of response to treatment in such cases is helpful in that it provides evidence to support the diagnosis of an underlying condition or pain type that has previously failed treatment.

If the pain has been worsened by treatment, it is important to know the nature of the exacerbation. Occasionally, pain is exacerbated by complications that can occur during the performance of an invasive procedure, or perhaps by a procedure that failed to achieve the success that was expected. Medications also may produce problems when allergies are present or when unexpected toxic reactions occur. These problems should be noted for two reasons: so that the problem does not reoccur as a result of reinitiating the offending treatment, and because some complications produce predictable problems that can be managed if recognized. An example of this type of complication is seen when nerve injury occurs in association with some chemotherapy agents used to treat a cancer. The resulting pain often is predicted and, when recognized, treatable.

A management history that summarizes the pros and cons of previous treatment is invaluable to the health care professional who is attempting to design an effective treatment plan. It allows the provider to utilize previously successful methods and avoid proven unsuccessful options. A management summary is also invaluable for the pain sufferer who hopes for rapid relief without significant complications.

## Are Any Co-Existing Medical Problems Present?

Co-existing disease processes and their treatments can have a significant impact on the management plan adopted for pain control. Due to the potential worsening of the pre-existing condition, the presence of some diseases precludes the safe use of certain forms of treatment frequently used to manage particular pain problems. For example, individuals who have had a history of coronary artery disease, a previous heart attack, or heart failure should not receive certain antidepressant agents (e.g., amitriptyline) in the management of their nerve pain because this drug may worsen the underlying cardiac condition. In addition, some medications given to treat pain can increase or decrease the effectiveness of other medications provided to treat another disease, or they may render another medication ineffective or toxic. Therefore, for safety, it is essential to be aware of ongoing disease processes and concurrent treatments to avoid unnecessary complications.

An important corollary to this observation is that certain treatment options used for managing pain may provide benefits that extend beyond the primarily desired effect. With a knowledge of concurrent medical problems, particular medications used for pain control may be chosen to take advantage of what would otherwise be considered an adverse effect to provide instead a beneficial response to the individual. For example, medications frequently used to treat neuropathic pain also produce significant drowsiness. When these medications are prescribed for someone who has insomnia, both pain relief and improvement of sleep are achieved.

A history of allergic reaction should be provided. Previous allergies to certain groups of medications and the lack of reaction to other groups can provide important warnings as to possible adverse effects that may occur when previously unused medications are being considered. Although not an absolute contraindication for the use of opioid analgesics in the treatment an ongoing pain complaint, any history of substance abuse—including illicit drugs, alcohol, and tobacco—is important to know. A prior history of substance abuse should alert the health care provider to enhance vigilance to reduce the risk of re-establishing a previous problem of abuse and to be aware of potential tolerance to particular treatment options. A history of tobacco abuse may well affect the rate or likelihood of recovery from a painful injury.

## How Has the Pain Affected the Levels of Functioning?

The success of pain management often depends on realistic expectations for the possible results and an appreciation for improvement throughout the course of treatment, rather than expecting complete resolution of pain as the only acceptable goal. Depending on the severity of the condition that underlies the pain, the likelihood of curing the underlying condition, and the time that the pain has been endured, varying levels of improvement may be expected.

For those who have endured many attempts at pain control with several health care providers and who have suffered for many years, the likelihood of complete elimination of pain is very rare indeed. However, with patience and proper comprehensive treatment, the vast majority of pain sufferers can realize significant improvement in their pain. The level of improvement is determined to a large degree by a combination of conditions. The first is how successfully an appropriate treatment regimen is identified. The second is the individual's ability to tolerate and participate in treatment. The third is how effective the treatment is for the individual being treated. Ultimately, however, success is determined by how the individual receiving treatment perceives the response. Much of what determines success depends on the degree to which pain initially controlled the patient's life when compared to the amount of control regained by the patient. To provide a framework on which to build, the pain sufferer should provide information about his level of functioning prior to the onset of his pain. If he was unable to play piano prior to developing pain, it is not likely that pain relief alone will make that skill possible. During recovery, it is important to identify the point from which one is starting and to set short-term goals that are likely to be attainable as benchmarks of progress during treatment. Perhaps someone's initial goal is to walk 50 feet, then 50 yards, then a mile; perhaps it is to return to part-time work and then full-time work; or perhaps it is to be comfortable enough to see a son or daughter graduate from college or get married. The goals should be realistic and especially important to the one trying to achieve them.

The psychological aspects of pain play a significant role in treatment failure and success. Problems such as depression (which is frequently present in individuals who have suffered pain for longer than 6 months), anger, irritability, and frustration that often lie unrecognized beneath the surface are conditions that perpetuate pain. For many who suffer chronic pain, an underlying grief must be dealt with in order to move on to relief. The grief is most profound because it represents the loss of oneself, one's identity, or an image of who one was meant to be. Along similar lines, consideration must be given to the fact that pain not only affects the person who feels it directly, but affects all individuals with whom the sufferer has contact—spouse, family, friends, and co-workers. Thus, the psychosocial concerns for both the sufferer and his social relations are important to identify and to address if the best results are to be achieved.

# CHAPTER 3

# The Multidisciplinary Approach—The Best Way to Treat My Pain

ONCE THE PAIN PROBLEM has been evaluated and a diagnosis has been reached, it is time to determine what options are available to best manage the condition. Most pain sufferers and, indeed, most health care providers consider pharmacologic options or medications as the primary, if not only, appropriate method for treating pain. Not surprisingly, because of the complex nature of pain, medications alone often are insufficient to provide complete or maximum pain relief. Indeed, chronic pain influences many aspects of an individual's quality of life, from basic functioning during work, recreation, and the activities of daily living, to mood, sleep, self-image, and behavior, to social concerns about marriage, family relations, sex and intimacy, and economic status and security. It is thus unreasonable to expect that a single medication or one mode of therapy could effectively manage all the factors involved.

The concept of a multidisciplinary or interdisciplinary approach to managing pain was championed by John J. Bonica, who had recognized during his experience in World War II that he was unable to provide adequate pain relief for many of his patients if he utilized only the methods afforded to him by his training in anesthesiology. He realized that health care providers who had been trained in other specialties and had managed pain for their patients could add a new dimension to both the evaluation and treatment of complex pain conditions that did not respond to his particular treatment. Although perceived by some to be more complicated and more costly because of the initial multispecialty evaluations and treatments, multidisciplinary team management of pain has proven to be more effective and less costly overall than when pain is managed by different specialists working independently. The concept of the multidisciplinary approach to pain management can be illustrated well when viewed for comparison with the story of the blind men and the elephant (Fig. 3-1). In the story, five blind men happen upon an elephant. Each evaluates a different portion of what has been found, and each comes to a different conclusion about what it is. Not until the men share their observations and discuss what they have found do they know that they have found an elephant. In a similar way, pain problems, when viewed from only one perspective, are often inadequately evaluated, infrequently or inaccurately identified, and incompletely managed. The multidisciplinary approach results in a better return to functioning, less suffering, and reduces the overall risk of developing a life-long problem. The goal of the multidisciplinary team, therefore, is to identify which of the many treatments are likely to be effective and to determine when each should be implemented to provide the best care.

Multidisciplinary teams are composed of health care professionals, all of whom understand that pain is a multifaceted entity that reduces an individual's quality of life. They share a desire to help the pain suf-

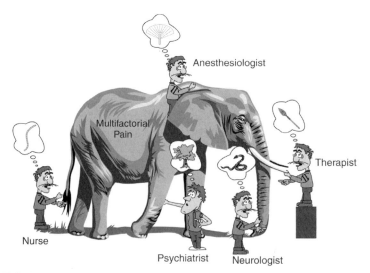

**FIGURE 3-1**

Five blind men and the elephant. (Modified from John Godfrey Saxe, 1816-1887.)

ferer decrease the burden of pain, using the tools of their special areas of interest and training. Their first goal of treatment is to identify and manage the condition responsible for producing the pain. Because treatment of the underlying cause for the pain in most instances will eliminate or significantly reduce the perceived pain, primary-care physicians are perhaps the best choice for coordinating the care provided. Their general knowledge enables them to understand an individual's overall medical condition, and they are best trained to monitor and predict how treatment options designed to improve a specific body system may influence medical well-being. Physician specialists in many areas, however, may be necessary and should be considered early for proper assessment and treatment, especially when pain problems involve particular body systems or diseases such as arthritis (rheumatologist), cancer (oncologist), diabetes (internist), or neurodegenerative disease (neurologist and physiatrist), or require specialized procedures such as setting a broken bone (orthopedist), removal of an inflamed appendix (surgeon), or local analgesia for delivery of a baby (anesthesiologist).

The second goal of the pain management team, one often overlooked by those less knowledgeable about pain, is to provide adequate and appropriate pain relief while the primary condition is being treated. It is not sufficient to rely on treatment of the cause of pain alone to provide pain relief. If pain is managed during primary treatment, the pain sufferer will have a better quality of life, will be more likely to accept necessary testing for diagnosis and management, and may be more compliant with treatment of their disease. Many people fear the pain associated with diagnostic testing and treatment, and often decline to pursue evaluation for that reason alone. Many of us would prefer not to visit the dentist for routine evaluations because of painful experiences that were part of our past, or we are uncomfortable visiting a physician because we recall the shots received from the doctor when we were children. Although many of the pain problems may be adequately managed by the general internist or system specialists, when individuals continue to complain of discomfort after initial attempts at pain control have failed, physicians who specialize in pain management may be able to offer a greater spectrum of options.

Psychological factors that can either amplify or perpetuate pain and may often impede its treatment are best evaluated and managed by psychiatrists and psychologists. These specialists observe behavior daily, and understand how coping skills and defense mechanisms can influence pain perception. Through specialized treatment options, such as biofeedback, hypnosis, and meditation, psychological resources may be accessed and cognitive skills may be enabled to improve pain control.

In practice, the physician's role is focused and relatively limited. The pain sufferer may see his treating physician only intermittently and for short periods. Nurses, therapists, and other allied health professionals, however, usually spend more time with patients, and they have a better opportunity to observe how pain impairs function and influences quality of life, and how treatments are being tolerated. Caring allied health professionals are therefore an essential component of a successful multidisciplinary team, because they provide both specialized education and treatment for reducing pain during activities of daily living and are well-positioned to monitor the responses to treatment initiated by other members of the team.

The efficient functioning of the pain management program does not solely rest on the efforts of the highly visible, "hands-on" health care providers. Behind-the-scenes support from pharmacists with knowledge of alternative medication options and drug interactions and social workers who can arrange access to community resources for providing care make it possible to shift pain management from the hospital and clinic setting to the individual's home and office. The coordination of available resources offers the most effective opportunity to achieve the most complete evaluation of a painful condition, treat the underlying cause of the pain, and provide adequate pain relief while treating the primary disease.

CHAPTER 4

# The Anatomy of Pain—
# The Basis for Selecting
# Treatment Options

DURING THE PAST DECADE, a significant increase has occurred in our knowledge about how pain is perceived, transmitted, and processed. With this improved understanding of the basic mechanisms responsible for processing pain has come the realization that medications previously not considered for pain control may have pain-relieving properties. These medications are called *adjuvant medications* rather than analgesics, because they were designed to treat another medical condition. These medications have an *analgesic* (pain-relieving) effect because the mechanisms through which they produce their intended effect also influence the pain processing pathways. This realization has led us to modify our basic approach for evaluating and treating pain. Instead of primarily treating the disease while secondarily managing the accompanying pain with analgesics alone, we now recognize that pain itself is a disease process manifested similarly in a variety of disease states. As such, pain is now viewed as a significant component of a patient's complaint, and it should be treated with attention equal to that given the underlying disease. By recognizing the similarities in pain symptoms across a variety of medical conditions, effective treatment plans can be designed to target pain processing mechanisms, thus providing adequate pain relief while treating the underlying disease.

From the perspective of the health care provider, it is no longer acceptable to assume that all pain is the same and that treatment with analgesic medications alone is appropriate for good pain management. From the perspective of the person experiencing pain, who may be asked to take a wide variety of medications, it is important to understand the rationale for the choice of these medications, especially for those not obviously associated with pain control. As a result of such understanding, compliance with the treatment regimen and ultimately improved success in reducing pain is more likely to be achieved.

This chapter briefly summarizes basic information about the anatomy that underlies our perception, modulation (adjustment), and transmission of a noxious stimulus. I also discuss how normal pain processing can be altered in different conditions, and how these alterations lead to the perception of pain. To appreciate the information given in the rest of this book, it is important to understand the locations along the pain pathways where medications are likely to have an influence on reducing the pain signal. In later chapters, reference will be made to the presumed sites of action for medications used to achieve pain control and to those sites that hold promise for the development of new treatment options. Much of the information that follows is complex, but time spent in reviewing it will be rewarded by a better understanding of why particular pain medications and treatments are selected to improve pain control.

## PERIPHERAL COMPONENTS OF THE NORMAL PAIN PATHWAY

Our ability to explore and evaluate our environment through touch is provided by special nerve cells called *sensory neurons*. The cell bodies of the sensory neurons, which are responsible for maintaining the functional integrity of the cell, are located adjacent to the spinal cord and brainstem in collections of nerve cells called *ganglia*. Ganglia are protected by the bony elements of the vertebral column that surround the brain and spinal cord; the central nervous system (CNS). A portion of the sensory neuron extends away from the CNS through conduits called *peripheral nerves*, which connect with all organs of the body. These neuronal processes, called *axons*, convey information about the condition of the internal and external environment of the body wall and body cavities to the spinal cord and brain, where it is consciously perceived. In the brain, this information is compared with past and present experience to determine if this is a recognizable event, interpret it, and then generate a behavioral response.

The structure of the peripheral nerves varies depending on the specific sensory function they perform. Many of the receiving elements of peripheral nerves are associated with specialized nerve endings, such as those illustrated in Figure 4-1, that enhance their ability to receive particular types of sensory information. For example, the *spindle organs* found in muscles that are under voluntary control, such as the biceps

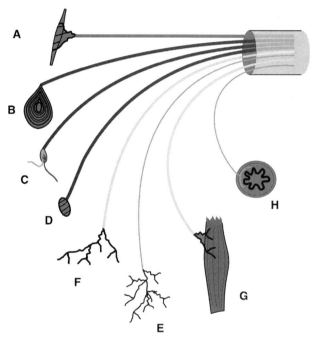

**FIGURE 4-1**

Sensory nerves and their specialized endings. Specialized peripheral nerve endings are associated with specific information that is received. Spindle organs (A) detect voluntary muscle stretch, Pacinian corpuscles (B) detect vibration, Merkel cells (C) detect light touch, Meissner's corpuscles (D) detect pressure, and free nerve endings (E) detect noxious stimuli. The specialized nerve endings are associated with specific axon types, whose diameter and myelin sheath determine the rate of signal transmission. Ia afferent (A, most rapid conductor), A-β (B, C, and D), A-β A-δ (F and G), and C-fibers (E and H, slowest conductor) are illustrated in association with their specialized nerve endings.

in the arm, are optimally constructed to detect fine differences in muscle stretch. Signals generated in those nerves having these specialized endings are responsible for the corrective contraction of the stretched muscle so that the appropriate muscle length and tension is maintained. The system of nerves associated with the spindle organs is tested when a tendon reflex (knee jerk) is elicited by a physician during an examination. In contrast, *Golgi tendon organs,* which are located in the tendons of these same voluntary muscles. are designed to detect levels of contraction or stretching force just below a force that would injure the muscle. When such a force is generated, a sensory signal is immediately transmitted that results in blocking further muscle contraction, thereby preventing injury to the muscle and its tendon. Other nerves that transmit information about very light touch, vibration, and position sense also are associated with specialized nerve endings. Unlike the nerves having specialized endings, those neurons that respond to stimuli of sufficient intensity to potentially produce tissue injury make direct contact with all peripheral organs of the body without the benefit of an otherwise specialized structure. The pain signals are generated in these free nerve endings in response to noxious chemical, thermal, or mechanical stimulation.

Nerves not only differ in the way they terminate in various body structures, they differ also in the information they convey and how that information is conducted. Impulses generated at the peripheral nerve endings in the body wall are passed to the axon. Those axons that monitor muscle stretch and tension are associated with nerve cells that require the least amount of stimulation to generate a sensory signal. These axons are the largest in diameter and conduct impulses most rapidly. The somewhat smaller neurons of the *A-beta* (β) *system* convey information more slowly and monitor non-noxious, tactile stimulation from very small body regions. Noxious stimulation is conveyed by two distinct axon systems having the smallest diameter, the *A-delta* (δ) *system* and the *C-fiber system.* The A-δ system monitors relatively small body regions, precisely localizes the noxious stimulus, and conveys this information rapidly to the CNS so that an appropriate and timely avoidance response can be made to prevent further injury.

In contrast to the A-δ system, the C-fiber system monitors relatively large body areas. The information conveyed by the C-fibers is conducted more slowly and is less clearly defined. Most of us who have had the experience of striking a finger with a hammer while trying to drive a nail are well aware of the existence of these two systems. The A-δ system conveys the immediate, precisely localized pain that stops us from applying additional force to the hammer strike. Minutes later, the C-fiber system begins to send a more diffuse, throbbing, and persistent signal that decreases our desire to use the finger until the wound has healed, thereby decreasing the likelihood of worsening the injury.

The ability of an axon to rapidly conduct a signal is related not only to the diameter of the axon, but to the presence of a multilayered, insulating substance called *myelin*. Myelin is produced by specialized supporting cells called *Schwann cells*, which are aligned along the entire path of neuronal axons. When Schwann cells are associated with large-diameter axons, they produce a cell membrane that wraps around each axon in a jelly roll fashion. The resulting myelin sheath insulates each axon from its neighbors in a fashion similar to the insulation on individual wires in an electrical cable. Unlike the insulation on electrical cable, however, the insulating cover of the myelin sheath is interrupted at intervals along the course of the axon. The gaps in the myelin cover are called *nodes of Ranvier* and correspond to "excitable" areas of the axon. The property of excitability is conveyed to the axonal membrane by the presence of channels or pores that open and close in response to a stimulus. When the channels are open, electrically charged sodium ions are allowed to enter the nerve cell, resulting in a change in the electrical charge across the axonal membrane (Fig. 4-2). The change in electrical charge or *depolarization* stimulates the opening of additional channels in a sequential fashion, like the fall of dominos in a line. This causes the conduction of a nerve signal or *action potential*. In myelinated neurons, impulse propagation occurs only at the nodes of Ranvier, where sodium channels are found in the highest concentrations.

Figure 4-3 illustrates how the spacing of the nodes of Ranvier allows for the nerve impulse to traverse the length of the axon quickly by "jumping" between adjacent nodes, thus effectively shortening the length of axon to be depolarized. In axons that do not possess myelin, as

A

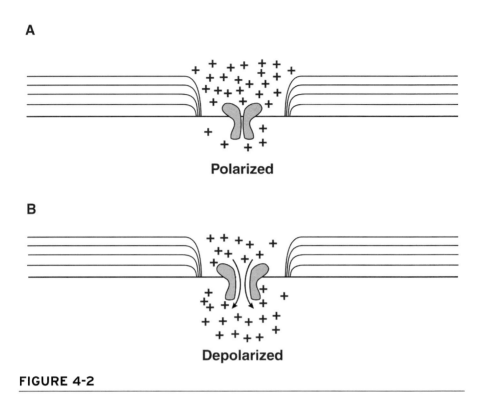

**Polarized**

B

**Depolarized**

## FIGURE 4-2

Charge distribution across: (A) a polarized (channel closed) and (B) a depolarized (channel open) membrane. + represents a sodium ion (charged particle). A representative channel is depicted in gray at a node of Ranvier between segments of myelin.

in the C-fiber system, depolarization must progress along contiguous areas of the axonal membrane, resulting in comparatively slow conduction of the signal. A simple example of the effect of an analgesic on this system is the numbing effect and pain relief achieved when local anesthetics are given by the dentist prior to drilling a tooth. The anesthetic blocks entry of sodium ions through the channels in the nerve cell membrane, thereby preventing the conduction of the pain signal to the brain.

Myelin may be disrupted when nerves are injured, which results in larger areas of excitable membrane along the course of the nerve. Due to the higher concentration of sodium channels in these damaged regions, nerve impulses can be spontaneously generated at these injury sites, resulting in more frequent pain signals being conducted to the

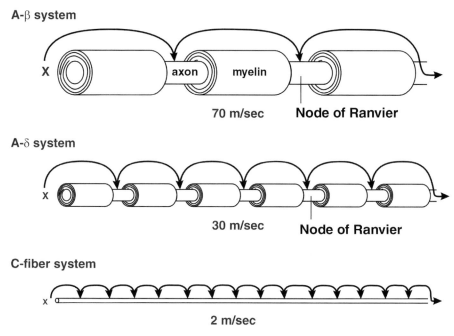

**A-β system**

axon
myelin
X
70 m/sec
**Node of Ranvier**

**A-δ system**

X
30 m/sec
**Node of Ranvier**

**C-fiber system**

X
2 m/sec

## FIGURE 4-3

Myelin, axon diameter, and conduction velocity. Conduction velocity is determined by the diameter of the axon and the amount of myelin present. The largest axons have more myelin. There is a greater distance between the nodes of Ranvier. Impulses "jump" between adjacent nodes of Ranvier, bypassing segments of the axonal membrane along the course of the axon like an express train en route to the spinal cord. These axons conduct impulses at the highest velocity. The slowest conducting axons are the smallest in diameter, do not possess a myelin sheath, and do not have nodes of Ranvier. The course to the spinal cord is traversed more slowly because, like a train making local stops, the nerve impulse (wave of depolarization) must spread to immediately adjacent portions of the membrane.

spinal cord and brain. An understanding of this feature of nerve functioning and injury has led to the clinical use of medications that block sodium channels to treat pain associated with nerve injury.

## SPINAL COMPONENTS OF THE NORMAL PAIN PATHWAY

As the peripheral nerves approach the spinal cord, the axons carrying sensory information to the CNS split away from the axons in the main

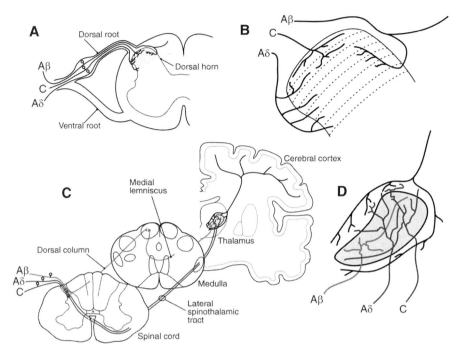

## FIGURE 4-4

Distribution of pathways involved in transmitting pain from peripheral nerves to higher levels of the brain for processing. Panel A depicts sensory nerves passing through dorsal roots en route to points of termination in the dorsal horn of the spinal cord and medulla (brain stem). Specific fiber types terminate in different portions of the dorsal horn as illustrated in Panel B. Signals effectively relayed in the spinal cord and brain stem course along specific pathways in the central nervous system, illustrated in Panel C, (dorsal column/medial lemniscus and lateral spinothalamic tract) and terminate in precise topographic fashion in the thalamus (Panel C and enlarged in Panel D) where the painful stimulus reaches conscious levels. Projections from the thalamus connect with areas of cerebral cortex (Panel D) where further analysis and association with past experience is made.

nerve trunk that carries both sensory information toward and motor information away from the CNS. The sensory axons travel toward the spinal cord in a bundle called a *dorsal root*. The cell bodies of the sensory nerves are clustered together at a point along the course of the dorsal root, in a collection of nerve cells called a dorsal root ganglion. The sensory axons continue past the *dorsal root ganglion* to enter the spinal cord.

Upon entering the spinal cord, the axons ascend toward the brain and enter the gray matter of the spinal cord at an area called the *dorsal horn* (Fig. 4-4). Like the passing of a baton in a relay race, in the dorsal horn, nerve impulses are passed from the peripheral nerve to the next relay neuron in the chain through the release of chemical substances called *neurotransmitters*. Neurotransmitters are stored within small packages called *vesicles* in the nerve terminal. The complex structures formed in the dorsal horn by the peripheral nerve terminal and the receiving cell is called the *synapse*.

For the neurotransmitter to be released from a nerve terminal, the transmitter must be available, calcium must be present in the terminal, and the terminal membrane must be activated. When the signal reaches the nerve terminal, calcium is allowed to enter through channels that open when a change in electrical charge is detected. In the presence of calcium, vesicles containing neurotransmitter fuse with the cell membrane of the nerve terminal. The neurotransmitter is released into the space between the two cells—the synaptic cleft. Released neurotransmitters recognize specific sites or receptors on the relay cell and, through an interaction resembling a lock and key, alter the membrane properties of the receiving neuron, thus enabling the cell to fire and conduct an impulse of its own (Fig. 4-5).

The impulse that ultimately leaves the dorsal horn is transmitted along complex pathways through the spinal cord and brainstem. It terminates on a collection of neurons in the *thalamus*, a part of the brain that serves as the major relay station for all information coming from the body en route to the *cerebral cortex*. In the cerebral cortex, sensory stimuli are analyzed and compared with memories of past experience and emotional states; this contributes to the modification of behavior. Axons that leave the cortex to return to the thalamic relay nuclei can increase or decrease the level of thalamic activity and thus modify the level of pain perceived and reported.

The dynamic relationship between the thalamic neurons and the cortical modulating cells determines the intensity of the unique painful experience perceived by each individual at any moment in time. Like setting a thermostat, the balance between excitation and inhibition that

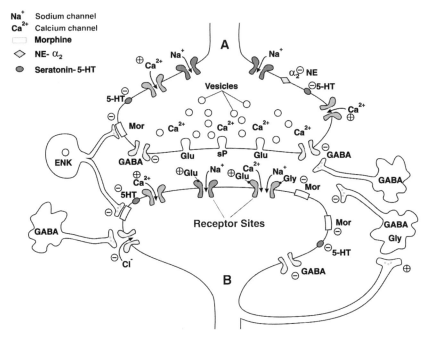

**FIGURE 4-5**

Peripheral nerve terminal (A) synapses with relay neuron (B). When a wave of axonal depolarization arrives at the nerve terminal via sodium channel (Na$^+$) activation, voltage-gated calcium channels open allowing calcium ions (Ca$^{2+}$) into the terminal. Calcium ions enable vesicles that contain neurotransmitter (glutamate, Glu; substance P, sP) to fuse with the terminal membrane, releasing their contents into the space between the afferent terminal and the relay neuron, the synaptic cleft. The neurotransmitters recognize and attach to receptor sites on the relay cell membrane. Channels open in the relay cell membrane, allowing sodium and calcium to enter. The relay cell is depolarized, generating an impulse that is transmitted to the next nerve cell in line. The release of neurotransmitter from the peripheral nerve terminal and the depolarization of the relay cell membrane may be modified in the presence of chemicals such as serotonin (5-HT), norepinephrine (NE), enkephalons (ENK), GABA, and glycine (Gly) that are released by neurons of the central nervous system that terminate in the dorsal horn of the spinal cord. These chemicals recognize receptors on the afferent terminal or relay cell membrane thereby increasing or decreasing (modulating) impulse conduction. The receptors can be influenced positively or negatively through the administration of medications that act directly on the modulating receptors (morphine, Mor) or indirectly by altering the activity of nerve cells that naturally release the modulating neurotransmitters. (Modified from Figure 6.3 in *Textbook of Pain*, Fourth Edition by Patrick D. Wall and Ronald Melzack, 1999. Reprinted with permission from Elsevier.)

sets the level of activity in the pain-processing thalamic neurons can be modified by varying the amount and type of stimulation that terminates on relay neurons of the CNS, either through changes in normal neuronal function associated with disease processes or by modifying function through the use of medications.

Not all nerve terminals and the neurotransmitters they release stimulate the firing of the neuron on which they terminate. Some neurons normally found within the dorsal horn of the spinal cord or in areas of the brainstem release neurotransmitters that inhibit or reduce the likelihood that the relay neuron will fire and conduct an impulse to the next stage in processing. In the example given earlier—hitting one's finger with a hammer—most people have noticed that, in addition to expressing some verbal form of discontent, the injured finger is often shaken, rubbed, or placed in cold water in an attempt to reduce the pain. In so doing, the A-β fibers that convey information about non-noxious, light touch are stimulated. In addition to transmitting information about the painless stimulus to the brain, the terminals of these neurons also stimulate the firing of dorsal horn neurons that inhibit the firing of the neurons that relay the pain signal to the thalamus. Like dropping a baton in a relay race, the reduction in pain-signal transfer from the peripheral nerves to those relay neurons in the dorsal horn that project to the pain processing neurons of the thalamus results in a decreased intensity of the pain perceived in the injured finger during the period of rubbing, shaking, or cooling.

The effective transfer of pain signals also can be modified by those neurons in the CNS responsible for restoring the monitoring system to optimum levels of function. This is done in anticipation of additional need for warning as well as to modify behavior to reduce injury and promote survival. This function is built into the nervous system. At the level of the spinal cord, nerve cells located in the dorsal horn are activated when a signal triggered by a noxious stimulus is transmitted to a relay neuron. These nerve cells send signals back to the relay neuron to inhibit further activity, thus reducing the likelihood that multiple impulses, which could exaggerate the original signal, are sent on for higher levels of analysis.

A higher-level system for setting the level of noxious-stimulation monitoring is also found in nuclei located in areas of the brain called the *hypothalamus* and the *brainstem*. The hypothalamus monitors basic body functions such as thirst, hunger, satiety, sexual function, blood pressure, temperature, and emotion. It maintains normal body function based on both conscious and subconscious information sent from the cerebral cortex and various body organs. The output from the hypothalamus in turn modifies the activity of those brainstem nuclei whose cells send axons back to the regions of the CNS that receive the original primary pain signals—the dorsal horn of the spinal cord. These brainstem nuclei, either through blocking the release of neurotransmitter or stabilizing the membrane of the relay neuron, reduce the likelihood that signals of a painful nature will be transmitted to the thalamus (Fig. 4-6). The connections effectively "reset" a system that has been activated by a noxious stimulus, or set the level of the system to receive the next signal based on a given body condition.

An example of this system at work occurs when pain from stimuli causing significant tissue injury, such as a gunshot wound, is not perceived during the highly emotionally charged periods occurring in the heat of battle. Norepinephrine and serotonin are neurotransmitters released from the neurons of these descending pathways to produce the inhibitory effect. Their effect is enhanced by many of the antidepressant medications used to treat pain. The output of the brainstem nuclei are normally modified through the activity of opioid-like chemicals called *endorphins*, which are naturally produced by the brain. In clinical practice, their activity is influenced by opioid medications.

After an injury, it is important to be aware of the area that has been injured so as not to subject it to further trauma, which may exacerbate the problem. Neural mechanisms that increase sensitivity in an injured region enhance vigilance of the wound during healing and aid in recovery. Repetitive firing of C-fibers produces a gradual increase in the perception of a stimulus irrespective of an increase in its intensity (see Fig. 4-7). This phenomenon, called *wind-up*, effectively increases the likelihood that a stimulus will be relayed to levels of cognitive perception through a sensitization of relay neurons in the dorsal horn of the spinal

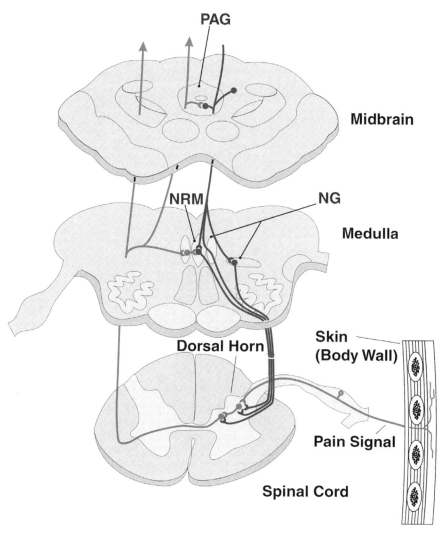

PAG

Midbrain

NRM

NG

Medulla

Dorsal Horn

Skin
(Body Wall)

Pain Signal

Spinal Cord

**FIGURE 4-6**

Descending systems modify pain signals as they enter the dorsal horn of
the spinal cord. Ascending pain pathways conveying noxious information
to the thalamus are depicted in gray. Descending pathways originating in
the hypothalamus, periaqueductal grey (PAG), nucleus raphe magnus
(NRM), and nucleus gigantocellularis (NG) are depicted in black. Like a filtering system, the descending projections decrease the amount of noxious
signal that is allowed to reach the thalamus through the dorsal horn of
the spinal cord. The filtering effect of this system is increased by using tricyclic antidepressant medications. Modified from M.J. Cousin and P.O.
Bridenbaugh, 1998. [Fig. 19-8, Wall/Melzack; *Textbook of Pain*].

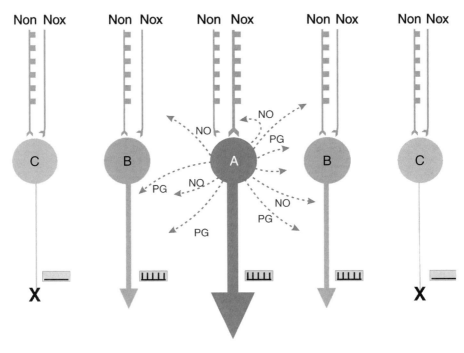

**FIGURE 4-7**

Central sensitization enhances the transmission of a pain signal. When pain signals (NOX) repeatedly cause relay neurons to fire (arrowhead), chemicals, such as prostaglandins (PG) and nitric oxide (NO) are released from the relay neuron (A) as illustrated in Figure 4-11. PG and NO make nearby relay neurons (B) more sensitive. Sensitized neurons can generate a pain signal (arrowhead) in response to non-noxious (NON) stimuli. By contrast, non-sensitized neurons (C) do not generate pain signals (X) when stimulated by non-noxious stimuli.

cord. The stage for repetitive firing is set by a process of peripheral sensitization, in which changes in injured tissue increase the likelihood that a warning signal will be generated in a primary afferent nerve cell.

## Pathway Alterations in Nociceptive Injury

For optimum survival, it is important to restore an area of injury as closely as possible to its normal structure and function. In some animals, regeneration allows for complete and accurate replacement of the injured body part and restoration of function. In humans, however, regeneration is limited, and repair is the primary form of healing. Repair entails the removal of dead tissue and any offending or foreign elements, followed by reconstruction of the injured tissue or replacement with a scar.

As illustrated in Figure 4-8A, when tissue is injured by a thermal, mechanical, or chemical stimulus, chemicals are released by local structures in the region. These chemicals stimulate increases in blood flow to the injured area, which brings cells that engulf and destroy nonviable tissues and infectious agents; increases levels of oxygen and nutrients necessary for repair; sequesters particulate byproducts of the clean-up; and removes the byproducts of metabolism in the form of carbon dioxide. This process of clean-up and repair is called *inflammation*. The chemical agents released during inflammation also serve to diminish further injury by lowering the threshold of nerve cells for generating a pain signal, thus making it easier to send a protective warning to the spinal cord and brain.

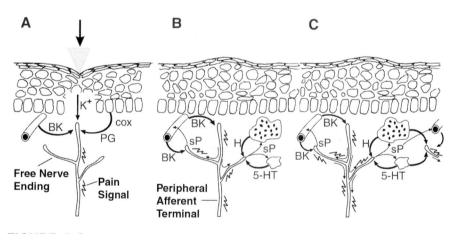

**FIGURE 4-8**

Inflammatory enhancement of the pain signal. Panel A shows that noxious stimulation (arrow) results in the local release of protons ($K^+$) and inflammatory chemicals, bradykinin (BK) and prostaglandins (PG). A pain signal is initiated and transmitted to the spinal cord. Panel B illustrates the nerve impulse as it also extends into the peripheral terminal branches of free nerve endings causing the release of neurochemicals, like substance P (sP), that stimulate the release of additional BK and other chemicals, histamine (H) and serotonin (5-HT). BK, H, and 5-HT make local and adjacent terminals more sensitive to stimulation and thus more likely to generate a pain signal in response to any stimulus (Panel C). Modified from M.R. Byers and J.J. Bonica, 2001. [Fig. 3-24, *Bonica's Management of Pain*, 3rd Ed.]

When a nerve impulse en route to the spinal cord from an area of injury arrives at a branch point in the axon (Fig. 4-8B), the signal splits and proceeds both along the intended route of transmission toward the spinal cord and to nearby terminal nerve branches. When the impulse reaches the free nerve endings, neurochemicals are released that further sensitize adjacent nerve terminals (Fig. 4-8C), potentiate the inflammatory process, and enhance tissue healing.

Because pain signals a threat to the integrity of at least some part of an individual, it naturally follows that a painful stimulus will set in motion a series of events that automatically prepares the individual for survival. This is the *fight-or-flight response*. These events involve the sympathetic nervous system (Fig. 4-9), a part of the nervous system that controls blood pressure, heart rate, breathing rate, and the volume of blood flowing to specific tissues. When this response is activated, more blood flows to voluntary muscles, heart, and lung, and less to the intestinal system and skin. Norepinephrine is the neurotransmitter released to produce these responses. When released in the vicinity of peripheral afferent nerve terminals, impulse generation is made easier.

## PATHWAY ALTERATIONS FOLLOWING NERVE INJURY

When nerves are injured as a result of cutting, blunt trauma, or compression, changes occur that allow nerve impulses to be generated at sites along the course of an axon, rather than just at the nerve terminals and synapses (Fig. 4-10). These abnormal generator sites occur where myelin is disrupted, thereby allowing extra sodium channels to be inserted into the unprotected axonal membrane as if it was a node of Ranvier. Because of this increased numbers of sodium channels, spontaneous channel openings allow the entry of sufficient sodium ions into the axon to trigger an impulse. The wave of depolarization proceeds away from the active site in both directions—toward the spinal cord and toward the body surface. As in nociceptive injury, when a nerve impulse reaches the free endings of the afferent nerve terminal, neurochemical mediators are released from the terminals, resulting in peripheral sensitization of the adjacent nerve terminals. As with normally transmitted

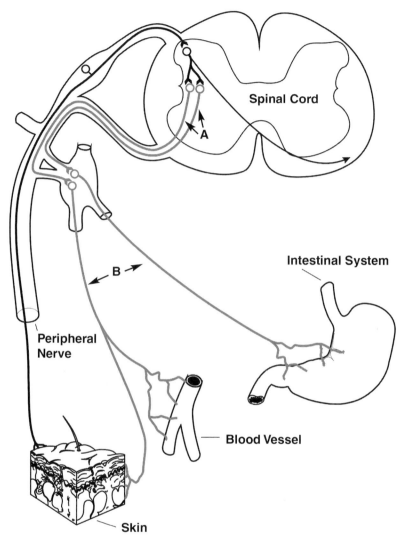

**FIGURE 4-9**

When a noxious stimulus enters the spinal cord, a portion of signal reaches neurons of the sympathetic nervous system (indicated by arrows A and B). These neurons send impulses back to the area of injury to regulate blood flow to the skin, and to voluntary muscles, the heart, lungs, and the intestinal system to prepare the body for 'fight or flight'. The neurotransmitter, norepinephrine, that is released at the peripheral sympathetic nerve terminals increases the sensitivity of peripheral sensory nerves to stimulation. Modified from M.R. Byers and J.J. Bonica, 2001. [Fig. 3-25C, *Bonica's Management of Pain*, 3rd Ed.]

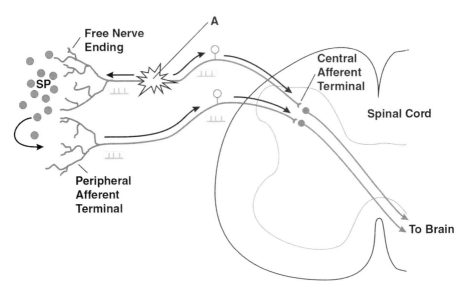

**FIGURE 4-10**

Ectopic firing of injured nerve cells and peripheral sensitization. When peripheral nerves are injured, nerve impulses can be generated spontaneously at abnormal (ectopic) sites along the axon (A). An impulse is transmitted to the spinal cord and brain in the normal fashion, but in addition, is transmitted peripherally to the afferent terminals. Chemicals, such as substance P (sP), are released and sensitize adjacent free nerve endings (curved arrow. Also see Figure 4-8). The sensitized nerve endings may then transmit a pain signal in response to a non-noxious stimulus. (Modified from Figure 5 in "Neuropathic pain: aetiology, symptoms, mechanisms, and management by CJ Woolf and RJ Mannion. Reprinted from *The Lancet* 1999; 353:1959-1964 with permission from Elsevier.)

nerve signals, those impulses that reach the spinal cord, thalamus, and cortex are perceived as pain in the region of the body served by the aberrantly firing nerve, even in the absence of a noxious stimulus.

Abnormal firing of this nature occurs in situations of toxic nerve injury associated with disease or drugs, as well as following traumatic injury to nerves and nerve roots in association with limb amputations and herniated intervertebral disks. Similar phenomena occur in association with spinal cord injury due to disease or trauma, with the perception of pain related to the area of the body served by the abnormally active portion of the nervous system. The behavioral response then is directed toward the area of perceived injury.

Persistent, spontaneous signals that reach relay cells in the dorsal horn of the spinal cord, and which continue for an extended period, activate processes that increase the sensitivity of the primary target neuron as well as neighboring relay neurons in the area. This process is illustrated in Figure 4-11. As a result, these relay neurons send pain signals more frequently, thereby increasing the intensity of the pain and the likelihood that the signal will reach conscious levels of perception. The process also

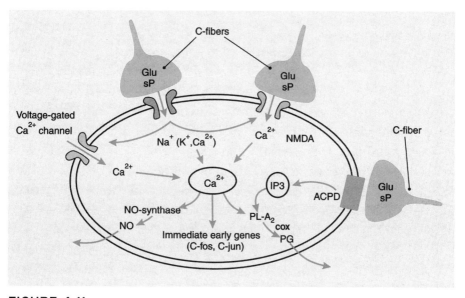

**FIGURE 4-11**

Making pain memories. Initial pain signals (C-fibers) cause the release of neurotransmitters, glutamate (Glu) and substance P (sP), from nerve terminals. Glutamate recognizes specific receptor sites on relay cells, and like a "key in a lock," opens channels that allow sodium to enter and depolarize the membrane. A signal is then generated. When stimulation occurs frequently, other specialized glutamate receptors (N-methyl-D-aspartate, NMDA) and voltage-gated calcium channels open, allowing calcium ($Ca^{2+}$) to enter. High levels of calcium inside the relay cell enable the production of nitric oxide (NO) and prostaglandins (PG). PG production is further enhanced by activation of additional specialized glutamate receptors (1-amino-cyclopentane-1, 3,-dicarboxylic acid, ACPD). When released from the cell, NO and PG sensitize locally adjacent pain relay neurons, making them more likely to generate a signal. "Pain memories" may be established if this process continues through the activation of immediate early genes that make the formation of new connections possible. Modified from H. Ollat and P. Cesaro, 1995.

sensitizes adjacent pain signaling neurons in the dorsal horn, enabling them to be triggered by non-noxious stimuli (see Fig. 4-7). If allowed to continue, in a fashion similar to repeating an address or a phone number, additional events are initiated within the relay neurons. This causes new neuronal circuits to be irreversibly established to allow pain signals to be more readily transmitted; that is, the brain learns to recall and experience pain. Clearly, a major goal of effective, early treatment for pain is to prevent this series of events from occurring and thereby preclude the development of a chronic pain condition.

In summary, the processing of painful signals within the nervous system involves many components that both sequentially and simultaneously process information in a fashion designed to enhance individual survival. Although the system provides many fail-safe mechanisms to ensure the integrity of the warning system to protect against serious injury, these same mechanisms may lead to problems and frustration in achieving complete or even adequate pain relief. To achieve the best possible treatment of pain, all components of the pain pathways must be considered as possible sources for pain generation and as possible avenues for achieving pain control.

CHAPTER 5

# Nonpharmacologic Options for Pain Management

IN TODAY'S SOCIETY, we seem to be conditioned to think that, when pain occurs, a medication should be available to produce relief. Yet, clearly instances occur when medication is not necessary to manage pain or is insufficient to produce the desired level of relief. In situations when acute pain related to a cut, burn, or abrasion is present, an immediate withdrawal movement occurs to separate the affected body part from the noxious stimulus. The withdrawal is usually followed by some form of verbal expression, repeated movements, or shaking of the affected part, and an attempt to redirect attention from the site of the pain by looking away. These behavioral responses usually reduce the intensity of the acute pain and, unlike medications, have little adverse effect. In chronic pain states, when medications are being used, we tend to forget these nonpharmacologic methods for decreasing pain intensity, or we limit their use and rely solely on "better living through chemistry."

Part of the reason for the under-utilization of nonpharmacologic methods is the lack of understanding that such methods are beneficial in producing a significant amount of pain relief. This misunderstanding may lead to the patient's belief that, if these methods are recommended by their health care provider, then the pain being reported is either considered insignificant or it is not considered a legitimate complaint. In other words, "The doctor thinks I am making it up" or "He thinks the pain is all in my head." This belief produces an obstacle that frequently defeats the potential benefit of nonpharmacologic means prior to their initiation, and it effectively eliminates these methods as valid options for consideration.

It is helpful to know that the development of many of the nonpharmacologic methods for pain relief are based on an understanding of the pain-processing pathways and have a sound physiologic basis for their effect. The cortical control of basal body functions that underlies the principles of yoga and meditation takes advantage of the descending neuronal pathways to reduce activity in the pain-processing neurons, thereby reducing the amount of pain perceived. When individuals are well-trained in cortical-modulation techniques, it is possible to reduce heart rate, alter respirations, and reduce or eliminate pain. Unfortunately, most of us are not well-trained in how to access our internal healing resources, and we view these responses with little credibility.

Nonpharmacologic methods for pain control should be considered for all levels of analgesic treatment. In cases of mild pain, this may eliminate the need for medication. For moderate to severe pain, nonpharmacologic methods may reduce the need for medication or may enhance the effect of medications that have been dosed to their maximum level of tolerance. Multiple forms of nonpharmacologic treatment are available. In general, noninvasive measures are better tolerated and have fewer adverse effects.

The *cognitive*, nonpharmacologic treatment methods attempt to modify activity in that portion of the nervous system that functions automatically to regulate the tension in muscles and blood vessels, control heart and breathing rates, and moderate intestinal activity. The *parasympathetic* portion of this autonomic nervous system is most active during the vegetative or rejuvenative periods of life and serves to enhance digestion and restfulness. In contrast to the parasympathetic nervous system, the *sympathetic* portion of the autonomic nervous system functions during situations of stress and prepares the body for fight or flight.

In most instances, a balance exists between these opposing systems for maintaining optimum function and survival. Pain is interpreted automatically by the brain as a threat to survival and therefore tends to increase the level of activity in the sympathetic nervous system. Other factors, such as past experience, unpleasant images, and environmental pressures, also can increase stress levels and, as a consequence, sympathetic activity. All these factors contribute to the level of sympathetic activity and determine breathing rate, heart rate, blood pressure, and sensitivity to noxious stimulation. If one can augment the activity of the parasympathetic nervous system by inducing a resting or vegetative mental environment through relaxation therapy, biofeedback, meditation, and guided imagery, many of the sensitizing mechanisms that increase the pain response may be reversed.

Cognitive techniques focus on determining how an individual perceives, interprets, and relates to a painful experience, so that negative conceptions and responses can be identified and monitored in the hope of modification. Some of the benefit of cognitive therapy may well be related to a sense of improved self-esteem that occurs when an individual perceives that his life is under his control, rather than being controlled by pain. Most of the cognitive methods rely on following regular protocols that become familiar and reassuring with time.

Anticipation of the unknown is one major factor that leads to increased anxiety and an amplification of the sympathetic nervous system activity. This is clearly illustrated in the creation of action, horror, and mystery stories for the cinema, in which skillful orchestration of the unknown is used to build emotional tension in viewers. The simplest way to reduce cinemagraphic suspense and the sympathetic response to a movie is to reveal the unexpected twists in the plot and the conclusion of the movie (although this usually is not popular with other moviegoers). A similar technique is employed clinically by providing education to the pain sufferer and his family as to the nature of the pain being experienced, the treatments to be considered, and the expectations for response, both positive and negative. The effect is improved by fully answering any questions that arise concerning the pain. All the information provided can be set into the context of the individual's past for a more comfortable clinical experience.

*Progressive relaxation therapy* employs a protocol in which the therapist guides an individual through a sequence of specific muscle contractions and relaxations. The individual is instructed to focus on the changes in sensation when the muscle shifts from the tensed to the relaxed state, on the pleasant aspects of the change, and on the differences in sensation between the two states. Utilizing this method, the individual develops an awareness of when muscles are tense, recognizes the difference between tension and relaxation, and learns to induce a relaxed state in tensed muscles.

When a stimulus is isolated, or attention is directed toward a single point of focus, all aspects of the physical being are drawn into the response. Distractions such as soothing music, soft colors, and pictures of peaceful scenery tend to draw attention away from the primary site of injury and may help reduce pain. In cognitive therapy, *meditation* and *guided imagery* attempt to redirect or disperse attention away from the portion of the body where pain is present, or in the case of a procedure, is anticipated. The individual is asked to think about something outside the body or to visualize being in a different place or time. Concentration on pleasant, nonthreatening images decreases anticipatory stress and anxiety, and reduces each noxious sensation to one of many images to be processed by the brain simultaneously, thereby reducing the significance of any one stimulus. Perhaps the most dramatic technique in the meditation and guided imagery spectrum is *hypnosis*. For those who are receptive to being placed in an hypnotic state, significant reduction of pain, even to the level of surgical anesthesia, can be achieved. Hypnosis has been shown to be effective in reducing acute pain associated with the surgical cleaning of wounds and the changing of dressings for patients with severe burns.

*Biofeedback* employs physiologic monitoring equipment to reinforce cognitive training. Normally imperceptible biologic functions, such as brain activity, muscle activity, or electrical potentials in the skin, can be monitored by electrodes placed on the skin. The changes in electrical activity picked up by the electrodes can be amplified and electronically altered to provide a signal that can be seen or heard by the individual being monitored. In time, the patient learns to recognize the sights and sounds associated with the relaxed state and, through association with different relaxation techniques, learns to generate the desired audio or visual pattern.

In athletics, it is well known that, for optimum performance, competitors must be well conditioned both mentally and *physically* if they are to succeed. Similarly, for success in pain control, both the proper mental framework and physical conditioning must be in place if optimum healing is to occur. It is well accepted that lack of physical activity leads to decreased conditioning and decreased ability to function. With respect to sports, we often are told to "use it or lose it." The longer one is immobile after an injury, the harder it is to return to functioning. Indeed, the loss of strength in supporting muscles places increased stress on skeletal supporting structures, with subsequent acceleration of wear and tear and increased pain. Current recommendations are to return to activity as soon as possible and, as tolerated, to progress steadily to improve strength, range of motion, and endurance.

The mantra of "no pain, no gain" is not helpful in the context of rehabilitative therapy. In practice, some fatigue is important and beneficial to enhance conditioning, but actual pain that produces a withdrawal response is likely to be detrimental and should be avoided. This probably also is true for sporting activities, yet athletes often are trained or conditioned to work through the pain, and they probably pay for that behavior in the future.

Following injury, it is important to determine the limitations imposed by the injury and to devise a plan of physical activity to maximize existing function, regain lost function, and minimize further injury, all with the goal of returning the individual to a state of self-reliance. Physical and occupational therapists utilize temperature application, manual methods, therapeutic exercise, and stimulation techniques to assist in achieving these goals.

*Heat and cold* are used to alter circulation around the site of injury and aid in healing while providing some temporary pain relief. The nonnoxious stimulation of heat and cold receptors can disperse the area of the pain focus and reduce the intensity of the pain at the primary site of injury. In general, cold should be applied soon after injury occurs. In addition to providing pain relief, blood vessels in the region constrict to reduce heat loss. As a result, swelling and bruising, which can lead to further tissue injury, is reduced below what would have occurred if left untreated. After the reaction to the initial trauma has stabilized, the application of heat aids in healing by increasing circulation to the injured area, bringing in oxygen and nutrients, and removing damaged tissue and fluid from surrounding tissue. These methods should be used in combination with other treatment methods, rather than as the sole method of treatment, because the effects are transient, and prolonged use can reinforce a dependant or *sick role*.

*Manual techniques* such as massage, traction, mobilization, and manipulation are used to reduce muscle tension, increase muscle length, enhance circulation, and increase mobility in restricted joints. In contrast to *therapeutic exercise*, manual forms of therapy are applied by the therapist and produce passive movement in muscles and joints. The passive forms of treatment are especially helpful when the patient has insufficient muscle strength or is so severely restricted that movements cannot be self-generated. Interferential stimulators also may be used in this setting to generate low levels of muscle activity and enhance tissue healing beyond the period when a therapist is available. When movement is possible, however, exercise should be initiated to improve strength, endurance, stabilization, mobility, and coordination. Therapeutic exercise also stimulates regeneration and revascularization in injured areas. The pain relief that ensues as a result of these forms of therapy may be further enhanced by a form of superficial stimulation called *transcutaneous electrical nerve stimulation* (TENS). This form of stimulation is designed to stimulate the same type of nerve endings stimulated when one shakes an injured body part after trauma. Unfortunately, although pain intensity decreases in the area of stimulation while the stimulus is being delivered, the beneficial effect rapidly diminishes when the unit is turned off.

One's ability to participate in physical rehabilitative activity depends to a large degree on the individual's level of pain during and after therapy. When pain levels are too high, the amount of meaningful therapy that can be tolerated is low, and the enthusiasm to continue decreases. Therefore, if advancement of pain relief is to occur, it is important to coordinate analgesic treatment in a regimen of *tolerable* therapeutic exercise.

Acupuncture involves the insertion of needles through the skin into tissues underlying points located along lines called *meridians*. Acupuncture is used for the treatment of various types of chronic pain, from headache and low back pain to arthritis and postsurgical pain.

Although many of the reports that support the use of acupuncture are anecdotal, and many reports are contradictory, some individuals clearly respond to this form of therapy. Treatment may be implemented with needle insertion alone or may be accompanied by electrical stimulation through the needle. The mechanisms through which acupuncture produces its effect are not entirely clear. It is probable, however, that when effective, the stimulation produced by needle insertion enhances normal pain-suppressing systems in the brain and reduces pain signals that would otherwise reach conscious levels of perception. Although relatively safe when performed by trained individuals, acupuncture is, nonetheless, an invasive procedure and not without risks. Infections can occur if aseptic techniques are not practiced. Needles may infrequently damage underlying nerves or blood vessels, resulting in alterations in sensation or bleeding into subcutaneous tissues. Acupuncture has been implicated in collapse of the lung. Although no absolute contraindications exist to the use of acupuncture, care is recommended when it is used during pregnancy and in individuals with epilepsy and cardiac pacemakers.

Finally, it is well known that, in order to maintain optimum health, individuals must *exercise* regularly, eat a healthy *diet*, and get adequate *rest*. These activities improve body functions, reduce stress, and provide a sense of well-being which, when present, is accompanied by lowered perceptions of pain. Although a healthy lifestyle is frequently considered only in passing when methods for managing pain are discussed, it is essential for the individual suffering chronic pain to follow these guidelines if healing or a reduction in decline is desired.

Pain itself, however, may decrease our ability to comply. Pain often is used as an excuse not to exercise, it frequently interrupts sleep, and it may either increase or decrease food intake. The stress of chronic pain often is reported as a reason for starting, restarting, or increasing the use of tobacco, which further impairs healing and the maintenance of supportive body functions. Therefore, a concerted effort should be made to maintain adequate nutrition and participate in regular, daily activity within a range that enables the patient to awake the morning after with no more pain than was experienced the day before. Regular activity tends to improve cardiovascular, respiratory, and gastrointestinal functioning, and it often improves sleep. These nonpharmacologic contributions to pain management are under the control of the pain sufferer and, when successfully applied, return much of the control of life to the individual, rather than to pain.

# CHAPTER 6

# Pharmacologic Options in Pain Management— Nonopioid Analgesics

WHILE EVALUATING AND TREATING the underlying cause of a painful condition, it is important for the pain sufferer's quality of life to provide concurrent pain relief. The goal in providing treatment is to achieve the greatest pain relief with the fewest medications possible, at the lowest doses necessary, without causing adverse effects. Although it might seem logical that a single medication would fit the criterion for the fewest medications, it is more frequently the case that the best treatment plans employ several medications given at low doses because of the numerous ways that pain signals enter the nervous system and ultimately reach conscious levels of perception. The strategy is designed to block the pain signal in different ways at different sites and produce better results with fewer adverse effects. This strategy is not unlike competing in a team athletic contest, in which winning a game depends on several individuals playing different positions with different assignments. If only one player is utilized in an attempt to defeat a complete opposing team, the likelihood of winning is poor.

In deciding what course of treatment is most likely to be effective, several factors are considered. First, what type of pain is to be treated? Nociceptive pain—the pain associated with tissue injury—responds well to typical analgesic medications or "painkillers" (nonopioid and opioid analgesics). However, neuropathic pain, which is associated with an abnormally functioning nervous system, is more effectively managed with medications that are not usually thought of as pain medications. These medications are classified as adjuvant medications; drugs with analgesic properties that were intended for treatment of another condition, such as depression, seizures, or hypertension.

Second, is the pain condition acute or chronic? Acute pain may be treated as necessary and only when present, but chronic pain is best treated regularly and on the clock to provide the greatest benefit with fewest adverse effects. The rationale for this approach can be illustrated by comparing treatment for the occasional short-lived pain as occurs in association with a headache experienced three times a year with the pain of advanced arthritis, which is always present. In the former case, it is neither reasonable nor prudent to take medications every day for a condition that produces discomfort for only a few hours a year. The potential for adverse events from the daily treatment in that case would outweigh the benefits achieved. However, in managing acute pain, it is generally better to treat early in the course of the pain and, if predictable, treat in anticipation of the onset of the pain. This method of treatment usually results in a more satisfactory response with less need for extended care.

In contrast, the goal in managing chronic daily pain is to keep the pain at the lowest level possible, because it is easier to manage low levels of pain. This approach is often contrary to the way most individuals have managed pain throughout their life. The pain sufferer often is reluctant to take medications regularly, believing that they may become addicted to the medication or that the medication may ultimately lose its effect or may cause other undesirable complications. In practice, the management of chronic pain on an as-needed basis can be likened to an individual who finds a small fire in a wastebasket. A small glass of water may stop the fire from spreading, but is not used because the fire is deemed "not that bad and will probably go away. Besides, I will probably need the water later." By the time the flames have engulfed the curtains and the wall, the glass of water is no longer effective, and the additional damage incurred from the fire hoses needed to extinguish the blaze can be extensive. Managing chronic pain on the clock ultimately utilizes less medication, is more effective, and is associated with fewer adverse events than treatment provided only as needed.

Third, what is the level of pain to be treated? As in performing any task, it is important to select the appropriate tools for the job. One would not usually consider using a sledge hammer to hang pictures on a wall, nor a wooden mallet to break up concrete. The selection of the appropriate tools or medications for pain management is guided by an analgesic ladder prepared by the World Health Organization (Fig. 6-1). Each step of the ladder corresponds to a range of pain levels, with an indication of the group of medications most likely to be required to manage the pain at each step on the ladder. The typical analgesic ladder has three steps. The first step corresponds to pain levels between 0 and 3 (mild pain) on a scale from 0 to 10. These pain levels usually are controlled with weak analgesic medications such as aspirin, acetaminophen, and nonsteroidal anti-inflammatory drugs (NSAIDs; ibuprofen, Naprosyn). The second step of the ladder depicts moderate pain with levels between 4 and 6. Pain at these levels usually requires stronger medications, on the order of the weak opioid medications, such as codeine and hydrocodone. The top step on the ladder corresponds to severe pain, with levels between 7 and 10, and typically requires the use of strong opioid medications such as morphine. In general, weaker and less-invasive options are tried before stronger, more invasive options are considered.

The final consideration in the selection of an initial treatment regimen is the current medication regimen. How long has it been in place,

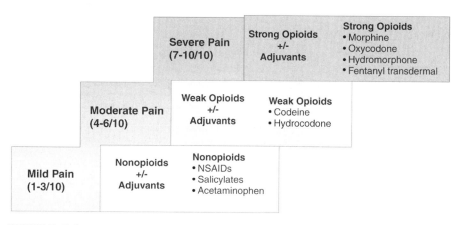

**FIGURE 6-1**

The World Health Organization (WHO) analgesic ladder provides a guide to initiating treatment that is likely to be effective for pain of different intensities.

and what has been tried before? The possibilities are great for selecting a medication that may produce good pain relief for individuals who are currently not receiving treatment or for whom a specific treatment has not been attempted. However, the options are more limited for those who have experienced multiple trials with medications or who are currently receiving medications to which tolerance may have developed.

## TOPICAL AGENTS

Weak analgesic medications are the best medications for the treatment of mild nociceptive pain. For localized and especially superficial pain, topically applied preparations are the best options. Many of these formulations employ local anesthetics that, when applied to the skin, are absorbed and block local nerve firing. Over-the-counter formulations of benzocaine or tetracaine are available for the treatment of pain related to sunburn. Antiseptic ointments that contain *lidocaine* or *Xylocaine* are available for the reduction of pain associated with lacerations and abrasions. (The local anesthetic lidocaine also is available by prescription in a patch formulation; this is discussed in a later chapter.)

Other topical formulations produce their pain-relieving effect through the depletion of the neurotransmitters released during the transmission of signals associated with a painful stimulus. These formulations contain *capsaicin*, which is the chemical found in chili peppers that produces the burning sensation experienced when eaten. This feature, while often desirable when mild and used in cooking, is the primary deterrent to capsaicin's use as a medication on painful areas of the body, because a similar warm to burning sensation is experienced when capsaicin is applied to the skin. For many, the burning is intolerable when applied to particularly painful regions and prevents the use of the drug. For those who can tolerate the treatment, however, the warm to burning sensation dissipates with repeated application (three to four times/day) over a prolonged period of time (4 to 5 months), leaving the region desensitized and less painful. Extreme care should be exercised when using this medication near the eyes and near sensitive tissues of the nose, oral cavity, and genitalia. The use of gloves is recommended.

Topically applied liniments and compresses that produce heat or cold also can be effective in reducing pain by reducing or increasing circulation to an area affected by strains, sprains, and overexertion. These formulations tend to effectively reduce or remove existing pain-producing inflammatory chemicals that make affected areas more sensitive to stimulation. Although heat and cold may be beneficial, care must be taken with those who have impaired sensory nerve function (such as diabetics) to ensure that tissue damage does not occur.

Finally, some preparations contain pain relievers that are more typically thought of as oral medications, such as aspirin. They are available for topical application and are used for localized pain associated with inflammation. These preparations are especially helpful for individuals who suffer from an inflammatory process like arthritis, but cannot tolerate anti-inflammatory agents when taken by mouth. The topical applications also may be utilized for the delivery of other weak analgesic and adjuvant medications that are not tolerated orally. Although not usually commercially available, preparations of specific drugs and drug combinations may be specially made by compounding pharmacists, who suspend prescribed amounts of these reagents in lotions, creams, or gels. These compounds can then be applied to localized areas of the body where they will be most effective. The duration of the analgesic effect for topical agents often is short when compared to orally administered drugs, on the order of 2 to 3 hours but, for some, the reduction in pain and the significant decrease in undesirable adverse effects often is worth the effort required to achieve relief. The cost of compounded medications usually is high and thus economically feasible only for small regions of the body, such as the joints of the hands and feet.

## ORAL AGENTS

For deeply located and more extensive pain, oral preparations are preferred. These medications fall into two general classifications. The first classification is represented by *acetaminophen,* which reduces fever and produces pain relief by an unknown mechanism. Although producing a mild analgesic effect, acetaminophen does not treat the inflammation that often accompanies mild nociceptive pain and therefore may be less effective than the second classification of weak analgesics, the *anti-inflammatory drugs*. Acetaminophen, however, is safer for use in those individuals with chronic gastrointestinal ulcers and hypertension. Its primary negative attribute is that a product produced during acetaminophen's breakdown blocks the effect of a liver-protecting hormone. The toxic effect occurs with increased frequency at doses that exceed 4,000 mg/day and is significantly enhanced when acetaminophen is taken in combination with alcohol. The toxic effect can lead to severe liver damage resulting in liver failure, cirrhosis, and death. Over-the-counter cold and pain-relief medications often contain alcohol or acetaminophen (Table 6-1). It is important, therefore, to verify exactly what medications, over-the-counter and prescription, the patient is taking before prescribing acetaminophen.

The anti-inflammatory agents include the steroid preparations, aspirin, and the nonsteroidal anti-inflammatory drugs (NSAIDs). These medications block enzymes that are part of the inflammatory process. Thus, they ultimately block the production of chemicals called *prostaglandins*, some of which increase the likelihood that a pain signal will be generated. Unfortunately, in blocking the undesired prostaglandins, the other prostaglandins, which protect the body in other ways, also are blocked, thereby increasing the risk of unwanted adverse effects. Steroids work at an early stage in the inflammatory process and at many sites within the body. Thus, they have more broad-ranging effects, but also have more potential problems associated with their use. Some of the effects seen with regular steroid use include a reduction in the immune response (which increases the risk of infection and some cancers), weight gain and altered weight distribution, thinning of the skin, alterations in blood glucose utilization, and decreased bone mineralization.

Aspirin and the NSAIDs have their effect on later stages in the inflammatory process than do steroids, and thus are more limited in both their positive and negative effects. They work by blocking cyclo-oxygenase (COX) enzymes. Prostaglandins that protect the kidney, stomach, and intestinal lining; play a role in platelet function (important

**Table 6-1**   What is in Your Medications?

**Selected Prescription Formulations**
**Containing Acetaminophen**
Darvocet®; Esgic®; Fioricet®; Midrin®; Norco®; Panlor®, Percocet®; Talacen®; Tylenol 3®; Tylox®; Ultracet®; Vicodin®; Wygesic®; Zydone®

**Containing NSAIDs**
Anaprox®; Ansaid®; Arthrotec®; Cataflam®; Clinoril®; Combunox®; Darvon-N®; Dolobid®; Endodan®; Equagesic®; Mobic®; Norgesic®; Percodan®; Toradol®; Vicoprofen®

**Containing Aspirin**
Darvon-N with ASA®; Hydrocodone with Aspirin; Lortab® ASA; Percodan®; Soma®Compound

**Containing Alcohol**
Atarax® Syrup; Bactrim® Suspension; Elixer Benadryl®; Chlor-Trimeton® Syrup; Darvon-N® Suspension; Dilaudid® Cough Syrup; Donnagel®

**Selected Non-Prescription Formulations**
**Containing Acetaminophen**
Alka-Seltzer Plus®; Anacin®; DayQuil®; Goody's® Powders; Midol®; NyQuil®; Pamprin®;Percogesic®; Robitussin®; Tavist®; TheraFlu®; Tylenol®PM; Vicks® 44M Cough; Vicks® Cold & Flu Relief Liquid and Liquicaps

**Containing NSAIDs**
Advil®; Aleve®; Anacin®; Ibuprofen; Motrin®; Orudis®

**Containing Aspirin**
Anacin®; Alka-Seltzer®; Bayer®; BC®; Bufferin®; Dristan® Sinus Pain Formula; Ecotrin®; Excedrine®; Goody's® Powders

**Containing Alcohol**
Cepacol® Mouthwash; Donnatal® Elixir; Dramamine® Liquid; Ephedrine® Syrup; Listerine®; Liquid Lomotil®; Micrin®; Scope®; Robutussin®; Tincture Paregoric®

for clotting blood); adjust blood pressure; and maintain pregnancy are not produced when NSAIDs are taken. As a result, the regular use of NSAIDs increases the risk for gastrointestinal ulcers, kidney failure, excessive bleeding, complications in pregnancy, and a reduction in the effectiveness of blood pressure control. In otherwise healthy individuals with post-traumatic injuries, however, the NSAIDs provide the greatest potential for benefit and are relatively safe for short-term use.

Recent investigations into the inflammatory process have shown that at least two genes play a role in producing the COX enzyme whose function is blocked by aspirin and the NSAIDs. The genes, *COX-1* and

*COX-2*, seem to be active at different times. They produce the COX-1 and COX-2 enzymes responsible for the production of different prostaglandins, all of which provide a protective function for the body. The COX-1 enzyme is always produced. The prostaglandins produced through COX-1 enzyme activity are responsible for the protective functions listed earlier (e.g., protection of kidney, liver, and intestinal lining, platelet clotting, etc.). In contrast, the COX-2 enzyme is only produced during inflammation. The prostaglandins produced through the activity of the COX-2 enzyme produce pain to alert the individual of current injury, which prevents or reduces further injury, and produce fever to establish an unfriendly environment for an invading organism. They also play a role in altering blood flow toward the injured site. This results in tissue swelling and the release of defending inflammatory cells from the blood vessels into the site of injury. A third gene, *COX-3*, only recently has been proposed. This gene or gene-variant may play a role in the production of fever, and it may be one mechanism through which acetaminophen controls fever, but its exact function in not yet known. The discovery of the genes for COX-1 and COX-2 in 1990 led to the development of a new group of anti-inflammatory agents that selectively inhibits the function of the COX-2 enzyme, thereby blocking the production of the prostaglandins that produce pain, fever, and tissue swelling without affecting the production of the prostaglandins that protect the stomach and kidney and that maintain pregnancy and platelet function. The hope for these medications was to reduce the adverse effects of the NSAIDs while maintaining the benefits they provided. In practice, the analgesic benefit provided by the COX-2 inhibitors was comparable to that observed with nonselective NSAIDs. In the first generations of these medications, the benefit for kidney protection was not found to be significantly greater than that afforded by the nonselective NSAIDs, but improvement in stomach protection was noted. No change was noted in bleeding time as a result of taking the COX-2 inhibitors.

A cloud of uncertainty has recently formed in relation to the safety of selective COX-2 inhibitors, particularly in regard to the potential for increased risk of heart attack and stroke in individuals who have chronically used high doses of these medications. Rofecoxib (Vioxx) and more recently valdecoxib (Bextra), were removed from the market when an increased incidence of heart attack was noted in individuals taking the medication. Although celecoxib (Celebrex) has not been found to have the same increased risk for cardiovascular complications, studies continue to clarify the position of COX-2 inhibitors in the prescribing armamentarium. The release of a new selective COX-2 inhibitor, lumiracoxib, has been delayed in light of current uncertainty for the future of this class of medications.

At present, it seems prudent to exercise caution when using these medications in individuals with a strong family and personal history of stroke, heart attack, and factors that increase the risk of cardio- and cerebrovascular events (e.g., smoking, diabetes, hypertension). In those with indications for an anti-inflammatory agent, however, the lowest effective dose of the medication, given for the shortest period of time necessary, should be used. Frequent monitoring for the development of cardio- and cerebrovascular signs and symptoms is essential.

Some additional features of the weak analgesics are important to note. First, these medications have a ceiling to the analgesic benefit that they will produce. Above a certain dose, no additional pain relief will be achieved using that particular medication. The risk of adverse effects, however, does increase with increasing doses beyond the analgesic ceiling, thus increasing risk without increasing benefit. The dosing of the weak analgesic medications should therefore be limited to the recommended maximum for pain control.

Second, many different preparations of weak analgesics are available. Because of their different chemical configurations, some agents may produce better pain relief than others. Of equal importance, some preparations may have equal benefit but produce different adverse effects, making one drug tolerable and another not. A corollary to this observation is that the benefit achieved with one medication in one individual may not be realized in another. Therefore, if one medication in this group is not tolerated or not effective, it is reasonable to attempt trials of other preparations before abandoning the drug class as a whole. The decision of which medication to use is based on its potential for benefit, the likelihood of adverse effect, frequency of dosing, and cost of the drug.

## Marijuana—An Old Drug in a New Role

Over several decades, much controversy has surrounded the legalized use of marijuana both for recreational purposes and as a therapeutic agent. Good evidence indicates that marijuana can be beneficial for the control of anxiety, nausea and anorexia, and pain, but therapeutic development has been impeded by concerns about its euphoric effects, its potential for abuse, and its usual route of administration. For years, an oral formulation of a synthetically derived delta-9-tetrahydrocannabinol (Marinol), the chemical naturally occurring in marijuana, has been available to stimulate appetite and reduce nausea in individuals suffering from AIDS and cancer and their treatments. More recently, experimental studies have identified at least two cannabinoid receptors on neurons and their supportive elements in many areas of the brain and spinal cord. These receptors are involved in the processing of a painful signal. It has further been shown that pain can be reduced when these receptors are stimulated. These studies have led to the development of a new marijuana-derived formulation that can be absorbed when applied under the tongue or to the lining of the mouth. The combination of delta-9-tetrahydrocannabinol and cannabidiol produces significant pain relief with no euphoria. It promises to be an important addition to our future armamentarium of pain-control medications.

Whenever nonopioid analgesics are used to control pain, success may be enhanced with the addition of an adjuvant preparation. As will be noted in a later chapter, adjuvant medications may potentiate the effect of the primary medication, may have a complementary analgesic effect through a different mechanism, or may produce an improvement in overall care due to the primary drug effect or a fortuitous adverse effect.

# CHAPTER 7

# Pharmacologic Options in Pain Management— Opioid Analgesics

S TRONGER MEDICATIONS MUST BE considered either when mild nociceptive pain is not controlled using weak nonopioid analgesics with or without adjuvant medications or when moderate to severe pain is reported. The medications represented on the higher steps up the analgesic ladder are the weak and strong opioid medications. The weak opioids are represented by codeine, propoxyphene (Darvon, Darvocet), hydrocodone (Vicodin, Lortab, Norco), and dihydrocodeine (Panlor). The prototype for the strong opioids is morphine.

Although opioid medications are the mainstay for the management of moderate to severe pain, they are unfortunately underutilized in the treatment of pain due to misconceptions about their use and abuse (discussed in the next chapter). Underutilization also is related to prescribing regulations that differ by the state or country in which they are prescribed. For example, prescriptions for opioid analgesics may not be written for a quantity that exceeds a 1-month supply, and a prescription may not be refilled without a separate written script. Second, copies of the opioid prescriptions, which often have to be written on special forms, must, at a minimum, be kept by the prescribing physician and the dispensing pharmacist. In some states, an additional copy of the prescription must be made and held by a state monitoring agency. Third, with the exception of an emergency, most opioid medications may not be prescribed over the telephone. A copy of the written prescription is required prior to dispensing. Fourth, if only a portion of a prescription can be filled either due to limited pharmacy supply or limited patient resources to pay for the medication, the undispensed portion of the prescription may not be filled without a separate written prescription. Finally, prescriptions for opioid medications may not be filled prior to the date indicated on the prescription, which can create problems when the prescription date falls on a holiday or on a day of the week when the pharmacy is not open for business.

In addition to regulatory barriers that are in place to reduce the likelihood that these medications will be used for purposes other than those for which they were intended, pragmatic barriers exist. These barriers are established by dispensing agents (pharmacies) as a form of self protection in a society in which these medications are obtained, disbursed, and used illegally. These barriers frequently result in inadequate supplies of medications in the pharmacies and, as a consequence, individuals who require the medications and who often find transportation difficult, may find it necessary to travel extensively to find a source for a sufficient supply of medication. This task must be done in person, since pharmacies, understandably are reluctant to provide information about their supply of controlled medications over the telephone.

Nonmedical complications not withstanding, when used properly for the appropriate reasons, most opioid medications provide good pain relief with no greater incidence of adverse effects than many other prescription medications. Some adverse effects occur so frequently, however, that they should be anticipated and managed preemptively. In any case, patients should be advised about the most frequent adverse effects and what should be done if they occur.

Constipation is an expected adverse effect when one takes opioid medications. It occurs so frequently that a bowel regimen should be initiated when opioid treatment is started so that more serious problems do not occur. The best advice for the management of opioid-induced constipation is to adjust the diet and use stool softeners and laxatives so that bowel regularity is identical to that experienced prior to taking opioid medications. A diet high in fruit and fiber, with increased fluid intake, may be sufficient. If not, stool softeners and mild laxatives, such as those listed in Table 7-1, should be used. Many individuals find that, after a time, one bowel preparation may lose its effect, requiring a change or

**Table 7-1**    Stool Softeners and Laxatives

| Laxative Formulations | How Effect Produced | Precautions |
|---|---|---|
| **Stool softeners** (Colace, Surfak, products containing docusate) | Add moisture to stool | Should not be combined with mineral oil |
| **Bulk-forming laxatives** (methylcellulose (Citrucel), polycarbophil (Fiberco), psyllium hydrophilic mucilliod (Metamucil), malt soup extract (Maltsupex)) | Dissolve and swell in intestine, lubricate and soften stool | **Diabetic caution**–some products contain sugar; should be avoided in individuals with narrowing of intestinal tract |
| **Lubricant laxatives** (mineral oil) | Coats and softens stool | Avoid in individuals taking blood thinners and those prone to aspirate; should not be used at bedtime |
| **Stimulant laxatives** (bisacodyl (Dulcolax, Correctol); senna (Ex-Lax, Senacot); sagrada (Nature's Remedy); casanthranol; castor oil; serotonin stimulant (Zelnorm) | Increases contraction of intestinal muscles | Use should be limited to 1 week; long-term use may lead to loss of colon function and worsening of constipation; castor oil should not be taken with food; can cause cramping, fluid loss and dehydration |
| **Saline laxatives** (Fleet Phosphosoda, milk of magnesia, magnesium citrate) | Draw water into the intestines increasing pressure and softening stool | Should be avoided in individuals with impaired kidney function, high blood pressure and congestive heart failure |
| **Enemas and suppositories** Microenema, Dulcolax suppository, Fleet Enema) | Cleansing sigmoid colon and rectum and mechanical loosening of impacted stool | Not recommended for chronic use; may cause fluid and electrolyte imbalances |
| **Synthetic sugars** (lactulose) | Draws water from body into the colon | May produce diarrhea, gas, stomach upset |
| **Opioid antagonist** (oral naloxone) | Antagonizes peripheral effect of opiate medications in the intestine | Abdominal cramps, diarrhea |

alternation between formulations. Tolerance may develop to many of the adverse effects of opioid medications, but seldom to constipation.

Other frequently reported adverse effects of opioid medications are drowsiness, nausea, vomiting, urinary retention, and lowered blood pressure and heart rate. These symptoms are not those of allergy, but indicate that toxic levels of the medication have been taken. The dose that produces these symptoms varies with the individual and may be severe. Toxic symptoms may occur at low doses, and most frequently occur in individuals who have not taken opioids previously. Withholding the subsequent dose or two and restarting treatment at a lower dosing level usually results in a resolution of symptoms and produces a desirable response.

Allergic reactions may occur with opioid use. These usually manifest as itching, rash and, when severe, difficulty breathing. Use of antihistamines may reduce these symptoms in mild cases, but the offending preparation should be discontinued and an alternative sought.

Respiratory suppression, euphoria, and mental confusion often are reported as adverse effects of using opioid medications. Because of the serious nature of these effects and the fact that they are frequently mentioned, many physicians have limited their use of opioid medications, and patients have been reluctant to take them. In practice, euphoria is infrequently experienced by individuals who are treated for pain using opioid medications. The pleasurable experience most often reported by pain sufferers is that of decreased pain rather than the "high" experienced by many individuals who take opioid medications recreationally. Respiratory suppression and mental confusion typically occur at dosing levels above those which would produce nausea and vomiting and are more frequently seen in individuals who take opioids regardless of their need to reduce pain (e.g., in drug abusers or laboratory volunteers), or in those who have other reasons for respiratory compromise (e.g., pneumonia). With respect to respiratory suppression, pain is usually a sufficient enough stimulator of respiration that respiratory suppression is not frequently seen clinically, outside of the immediate postoperative state. In the context of decreased mental abilities, high levels of pain often are sufficient in themselves to decrease concentration and the ability to do even simple mental tasks. In these cases, the pain relief associated with an adequate dose of opioid medication is initially likely to improve mental functioning rather than impair it.

## GENERAL PRINCIPLES FOR OPIOID USE

As with any medication, proper selection is important in providing optimum care with minimum problems. In general, opioid medications should be considered for moderate to severe pain of short (acute) or long (chronic) duration. For pain of short duration, such as that associated with minor surgical or diagnostic procedures (e.g., tissue biopsy or colonoscopy), a medication that starts to work quickly and works for a short time is preferred to something that takes hours to produce the desired pain coverage and lasts for hours after the procedure is over. For short procedures that are likely to be associated with moderate to severe pain and are usually followed by relatively short but variable periods of pain after completion (e.g., tooth extraction or fracture setting), a medication that acts quickly followed by one that is rapidly released but is relatively longer acting should be given. For pain that is likely to last for months to years, routine dosing of long-acting or sustained-release formulations is preferred, with additional immediate-release preparations available for treating the occasional acute exacerbations of pain that "break through" the routine coverage. Longer-acting medications provide greater uniformity of pain relief and decrease the frequency at which medications must be taken. This improves the likelihood that the medication will be taken as prescribed and decreases the individual's focus on pills to ensure a reasonable quality of life.

## WEAK OPIOID MEDICATIONS

As with most medical regimens, the adage of "start low and go slow" is appropriate for opioid use. Three opioid medications classified as weak opioids are frequently used in clinical practice. The first of these is *codeine*, the prototype of the weak opioid compounds. Codeine is a natural alkaloid derived from opium. It is approximately one-tenth as potent as morphine. It can be prescribed alone, but usually is found in combination formulations with acetaminophen. Codeine is used most frequently as a cough suppressant, for the management of diarrhea, for abortive treatment for migraine headache, and for moderate pain. Unlike the nonopioid analgesics, opioid medications have an advantage in that they do not have a maximum dose (ceiling) above which an increase in analgesic benefit can be obtained. Therefore, in principle, the dose of an opioid medication may be increased as necessary to obtain maximum effect. In practice, the dosing limit of opioid medication usually is determined by the onset of adverse effects. Most adverse effects occur because the medications used to manage pain circulate throughout the body and alter the function of tissues where the drug is not needed. As mentioned in Chapter 6, a second factor that limits the dosing of opioid medications is related to the potential risks for complications associated with the drugs that often accompany the weak opioid medications in combination preparations. The weak analgesic effect of codeine produces a third limitation in dosing: The number of pills necessary to produce significant pain relief is often very high and thus becomes the most significant factor limiting the use of this medication. In practice, 20 to 60 milligrams of codeine typically are used for pain control.

The second members of the weak opioids, *hydrocodone* (Vicodin, Lortab, Norco) and the closely related *dihydrocodeine* (Panlor), are formed by laboratory modification of the natural alkaloid (semisynthetic) of codeine. They are approximately one-third more effective in producing pain relief than is codeine. Hydrocodone only comes in combination formulations with acetaminophen, aspirin, or ibuprofen, which limits the dose that can be safely prescribed. Dihydrocodeine is formulated in combination with caffeine and acetaminophen. Because of the chemical modification, hydrocodone may be tolerated in some individuals who cannot tolerate codeine, and it is therefore a viable option for pain management for moderate levels of pain.

The third member of the weak opioid group is *propoxyphene* (Darvon, Darvocet). This medication is made entirely in the laboratory (synthetic), and is a derivative of methadone. It is less effective than codeine, having pain-relieving capabilities approximately equal to that of aspirin. It is available in combination with acetaminophen, which may be responsible for all the pain relief reported by individuals taking this medication. Propoxyphene should not be used in individuals with epilepsy or heart disease.

One additional medication, *tramadol* (Ultram, Ultracet), that typically produces pain relief at the level of a weak opioid, occupies a unique drug classification due to its mechanism of action. Similar to many other opioids, tramadol acts at the morphine receptor. However, unlike many other opioids, tramadol acts preferentially at the morphine receptor largely responsible for pain relief, and it acts less effectively at other morphine receptors that are more closely associated with the adverse effects. In addition, tramadol has effects similar to some of the antidepressant medications with analgesic properties. These antidepressant effects seem to contribute significantly to tramadol's pain-relieving action. The adverse effects experienced with tramadol are usually less than those experienced when taking other opioid compounds. This feature, combined with relatively low abuse potential, makes it an attractive alternative for pain control, prior to moving to the stronger opioid compounds.

## STRONG OPIOID MEDICATIONS

If the weak opioid preparations are ineffective for achieving adequate pain relief, strong opioids should be used. The prototype of the strong opioids is *morphine*. Like codeine, morphine is a natural alkaloid derivative of opium. It is readily absorbed into the body by all routes of administration—by mouth, injection, suppository, vein—and therefore may be useful in many medical conditions. In addition, morphine is available in many formulations that provide either immediate availability or sustained release. This allows dosing schedules to be tailored to accommodate the individual needs of the patient. Morphine is available in an immediate-release tablet or liquid that produces pain relief in 20 to 30 minutes and lasts for 4 to 6 hours.

If very rapid pain relief is necessary, an injectable form of morphine may be administered into muscle or vein to produce immediate relief. Intravenous doses of morphine are more effective than those given by mouth because, when injected, absorption from the gastrointestinal system is bypassed. When taken orally, morphine initially passes through the liver, where it is partially broken down prior to reaching its site of action. Thus, doses provided for oral consumption must be approximately three times larger than doses given intravenously.

Before additional doses are given, adequate time must be allowed for morphine absorption and for maximum blood levels to be reached. The *dosing* interval is necessary to allow an assessment of both the analgesic effect of the medication and the adverse effects that may be produced, prior to giving more medication that may add to either response. From the post-dosing evaluation, an estimate is made, based on the properties of the medication, of how much and how frequently the drug should be given.

Unfortunately, not all pain sufferers are able to tolerate morphine. For these individuals, the alternative strong opioid medications listed in Table 7-2 may be considered. Because of the difference in chemical structure, the drugs have different properties that may make them attractive alternatives to morphine. The decision of which drug to select is usually based on cost, convenience, and safety issues.

*Methadone* (Dolophine) is a synthetic, long-acting opioid medication with approximately the same potency as morphine. It is most commonly known for its role as a replacement for heroin in the treatment of heroin addiction. Methadone comes in liquid, tablet, and diskette formulations. As with other opioid medications, it has analgesic properties and is frequently used as an alternative to morphine when the cost of medication or opioid-induced hyperexcitability is an issue. Although methadone has a 25-hour half-life (that is, it takes 1 day for the body to eliminate half of an absorbed dose from the bloodstream), its analgesic effect lasts for approximately 6 hours. With regular dosing to ensure adequate analgesic coverage, slow elimination can lead to a delayed build up in methadone blood levels, with the subsequent development and escalation of adverse effects. It therefore is important to increase the dosing of methadone slowly, while monitoring closely for adverse effects. It is also important to note that many prescription medications may increase or decrease the breakdown of methadone, thus affecting the circulating drug levels for a given dosing regimen and making the dose either less effective or more toxic. On a similar cautionary note, concurrent use of some over-the-counter preparations such as St. John's wort, valerian, kava kava, gotu kola, and grapefruit juice may interfere with the effective use of the drug.

**Table 7-2** Opioid Analgesic Preparations Used in Pain Management

| Drug | Approximate Equianalgesic Dose (mg) | | Duration of Action in Hours | |
|---|---|---|---|---|
| | Oral | IV | IR | SR |
| **Weak Opioids** | | | | |
| Codeine (Tylenol 3®; Tylenol 4®; codeine) | 200 | 120 | 4-6 | N/A |
| Hydrocodone (Lortab®; Norco®; Vicodin®; Vicoprofen®; hydrocodone/APAP) | 15 | N/A | 4-6 | N/A |
| Dihydrocodeine (Panlor®) | 60 | N/A | 4-5 | N/A |
| Proproxyphene (Darvon®; Darvocet®) | 360 | N/A | 4-6 | N/A |
| **Strong Opioids** | | | | |
| Morphine (immediate release - MSIR®/sustained release - MSContin®; Oromorph®; Kadian®; Avinza®) | 30 | 10 | 3-5 | 12-24 |
| Oxycodone (immediate release - Roxicodone®; Roxiprin®; Roxicet®; Percocet®; Percodan®; Combunox®; Endocet®; Endodan®; Tylox®; oxycodone/sustained release - OxyContin®) | 30 | N/A | 4-6 | 12 |
| Hydromorphone (immediate release - Dilaudid®; hydormorphone/sustained release - Palladome®) | 7.5 | 1.5 | 3-6 | 24 |
| Methadone (Dolophine®) | 20 | 10 | 4-12 | N/A |
| Meperidine (Demerol®) | 300 | 75 | 2-3 | N/A |
| Oxymorphone (Numorphan®) | 15 | 1.5 | 3-5 | 12 |
| Fentanyl (immediate release - Actiq®/sustained release - Ionsys®; Duragesic®; fentanyl patch) | 0.1 | 0.1 | 0.75-2.0 | 72 |

(continued on next page)

**Table 7-2** Opioid Analgesic Preparations Used in Pain Management (continued)

| Drug | Approximate Equianalgesic Dose (mg) | | Duration of Action in Hours | |
|---|---|---|---|---|
| | Oral | IV | IR | SR |
| Levorphanol (Levo-Dromoran®) | 4 | 2 | 5-8 | N/A |
| **Partial Agonist Agent** | | | | |
| Buprenorphine (immediate release - Temgesic®; Subutex®; Buprenex®; Suboxone®/sustained release - Transtec®) | 2.4 | 0.9 | 6-8 | 72 |
| **Mixed Agonist-Antagonist Agents** | | | | |
| Nalbuphine (Nubain®) | N/A | 10 | 4-6 | N/A |
| Pentazocine (Talwin®) | 150 | 60 | 3-4 | N/A |
| Butorphanol (Stadol®) | N/A | 2 | 4 | N/A |
| Dezocine (Dalgan®) | N/A | 10 | 2-4 | N/A |

*Oxycodone* (Percocet, Percodan) is a semi-synthetic opioid compound that is one and a half to two times more potent than morphine. It is a short-acting medication that is available as oxycodone alone or, as hydrocodone, in combination with either aspirin, acetaminophen, or ibuprofen. Like morphine, the effect of the immediate-release formulation lasts approximately 4 to 6 hours and must be taken frequently to achieve adequate pain control. A sustained-release formulation (OxyContin) is available that releases oxycodone over a 12-hour period; it produces more uniform coverage and is more convenient to take than the immediate-release preparations.

Over the past few years, the OxyContin formulation has received significant negative coverage in the popular press due to problems most often related to the improper use or abuse of the medication. The problems surrounding the improper use of this formulation are unfortunate, because, for many pain sufferers, oxycodone is the only medication that is both tolerable and effective in controlling their pain. The publicity has created a stigma against its use and has made it more difficult to obtain for those who need it. It is important to realize that the sustained-release activity of OxyContin and its morphine counterpart MS Contin is achieved through special tablet design; this design is negated if the tablet is broken or crushed. By so doing, the entire dose of the tablet is made available immediately, which can produce the undesired toxic effect.

*Hydromorphone* (Dilaudid) is a semi-synthetic opioid that is six to eight times stronger than morphine. It is a short-acting agent whose primary benefit is that it can be administered by many routes (e.g., oral, rectal, intravenous) and is often better tolerated than morphine. It has been reported to carry a greater risk of developing psychological dependancy, although the actual risk is the same for all opioid compounds. In spite of its relatively high potency, only small oral-dose formulations have been available; thus, it is often necessary to prescribe large numbers of pills, at relatively high cost, to adequately control pain. This problem may be solved, since higher-dose, extended-release preparations are currently in development.

*Fentanyl* (Duragesic) is a strong opioid medication, approximately 100 times more potent than morphine. It frequently is used in its intravenous formulation for analgesic control around the time of surgery. It is available in a patch that is applied to the skin. The patch delivers medication steadily for a period of 3 days. This method of drug delivery is desirable for those pain sufferers who have difficulty swallowing and for those who find it difficult to take medications on a regular schedule. The medication is readily absorbed through the skin, and begins to reach effective concentrations 3 to 23 hours after the patch has been applied. It may take 36 to 48 hours before steady drug levels are maintained. The patch should not be cut or altered in any way to prevent compromise of the delivery system. It should be disposed of properly to prevent children and pets from potential injury that may result from inadvertent contact with residual medication remaining in the discarded patch. In addition, the fentanyl patch should not be used by individuals who have never taken opioid medications, because adverse effects, if they occur, may last for prolonged periods of time due to the depot of drug that persists below the skin and continues to enter the bloodstream after the patch has been removed. Finally, some people find that in warm weather, perspiration presents a problem for patch adherence and results in poor medication delivery. Occlusive dressings are available to minimize this problem, through the pharmacy or the manufacturer.

*Meperidine* (Demerol) is a short-acting, synthetic opioid compound that is widely used for acute pain control. It is approximately one-tenth as potent as morphine, and its pain-relieving effect lasts approximately half as long (2 to 3 hours). It is most often given by injection in the emergency setting to abort severe pain such as that seen in attacks of migraine headache or acute trauma. Although meperidine does have a role in the treatment of acute pain when a short-acting medication with less likelihood of intestinal spasm is desired, it is, unfortunately, all too frequently used for the management of chronic pain. When meperidine is broken down in the liver, a toxic by-product is produced that puts individuals at greater risk for developing tremors, agitation, muscle jerking, and seizures. The potential also exists for developing a fatal drug interaction when meperidine is administered in combination with monoamine oxidase inhibitors (MAOIs), such as isocarboxazid (Marplan), phenelzine (Nardil), and tranylcypromine (Parnate), that are used to treat anxiety and obsessive-compulsive disorders. The risk of these adverse events increases with the frequency of dosing, which is a potential problem when pain control is only present for short periods. The complications can be avoided by using longer acting agents, such as morphine.

One last group of opioid medications to consider includes buprenorphine (Buprenex, Suboxone), butorphanol (Stadol), pentazocine (Talwin), dezocine (Dalgan), and nalbuphine (Nubain). These are part of the partial *agonist* or *mixed agonist–antagonist* group. This group of opioid medications works through more complex mechanisms than those described earlier and simultaneously produces opposing effects on different opioid receptors in the brain. That is to say, they simultaneously produce pain relief at one site and block pain relief at another. For treatment considerations, this dual mechanism, distinct from other opioid medications, imposes a dose-ceiling effect so that doses above a certain maximum will not increase pain relief. Such medications are thus limited in the pain relief that can be provided. It is especially important for prescribing physicians and for individuals who have taken other "pure agonist" opioid medications (such as morphine, methadone, hydromorphone and fentanyl) for a long time to recognize the action of mixed agonist–antagonist medications and be aware of the different ways in which they produce pain relief. The concomitant use of mixed agonist–antagonist medications by someone who routinely takes pure agonist medications for pain control can rapidly produce symptoms of withdrawal.

CHAPTER 8

# Opioid Analgesics—
# Myth versus Benefit

ALTHOUGH OPIOID ANALGESICS are effective medications in the management of moderate to severe pain, they have been underused in the battle to control pain largely due to misconceptions about the dangers of these medications. This is not to say that opioid medications should be considered free of problems but, as with any prescription medication, if used appropriately, for the right reasons, and while taking precautions to limit adverse effects, a beneficial and desired effect can be achieved.

From the perspective of the pain sufferer, a reluctance may exist to take opioid medications because of the fear of addiction to the drug. This fear is coupled with the concern about experiencing the symptoms of withdrawal should they occur. Pain sufferers also fear that tolerance may develop to the beneficial effects of the medication so that, when a true need arises, the benefit will no longer be available to them. Further concern exists that the toxic effects of the medications will result in a decrease in the quantity, as well as a decrease in the quality of life. Finally, those contemplating treatment with opioid medications fear the social stigma of being viewed as weak, or worse, as a drug addict, by themselves, their family, many health care providers, and their friends.

Further impediments to the appropriate use of opioid medications are related to the misconceptions of the health care provider. A fear exists of producing addiction in those individuals for whom opioid medications are regularly prescribed. Indeed, many physicians who do not treat pain on a regular basis believe that patients who require a regular regimen of opioid medications for pain management are "addicted" to the medication and all too frequently refer to such patients as "addicts." Furthermore, little comfort is gained in providing opioid medications for the management of chronic pain due to a general paucity of training in the proper use of opioid medications and the assessment and management of the potential complications.

Finally, from the perspective of the health care system, inconsistent and often cumbersome regulatory policies are related to the prescribing of opioid medications, especially for the management of pain not associated with terminal disease. In addition, the often capricious meting out of sanctions related to perceived inappropriate prescribing practices result in a basic reluctance by the provider to prescribe. This confluence of circumstances leads to underutilization of the opioid medications and undertreatment of moderate to severe pain. Only through improved education about both the positive and negative attributes of opioid medications will rational thinking prevail and pain control improve. In an attempt to dispel some of the misconceptions related to opioid medication, I select and discuss some of concerns that are most frequently expressed in the context of my practice.

## WILL I BECOME ADDICTED TO THE MEDICATION?

It may be comforting to know that, although addiction is one of the potential adverse effects of taking opioid medications, the risk of becoming addicted to an opioid medication that is taken appropriately for the treatment of pain is very low. Indeed, the incidence of addiction to opioid medications used for the management of pain is less than 5%. This is not to say that physical and behavioral complications similar to those observed in addiction may not occur when taking opioid medications for appropriate reasons. These complications must be assessed and distinguished from other conditions that have similar physical and behavioral manifestations, and they must be managed appropriately. It is therefore important to understand the difference between addiction, dependancy, tolerance, and pseudoaddiction (false addiction).

*Addiction* is a psychological dependency on any substance taken for the psychological benefits that are derived, irrespective of therapeutic necessity and despite effects that are identified and found to be deleterious to the health of the individual. Depending on the substance abused—tobacco, alcohol, opioid medications, tranquilizers, or stimulants—*physical dependency* occurs in addition to the addiction. This physical dependency underlies the development of withdrawal symptoms when the abused substance is abruptly discontinued.

In contrast to addiction, physical dependency is an adaptive phenomenon in which cells of the body alter their normal function to accommodate for repetitive exposure to certain regularly taken substances. Because of the physical changes that occur, when the inducing stimulus is withdrawn abruptly, a period occurs during which the normal cellular function is reestablished, when the altered cells' function is poorly controlled, and the symptoms of withdrawal ensue. If treatment is no longer necessary, normal cellular functioning can be re-established gradually through incremental decreases in dosing, thereby preventing the abnormal cellular function and the development of withdrawal symptoms. Physical dependency is to be expected in individuals who take opioid medications regularly for the treatment of chronic pain, but it does not mean that, if and when the pain is no longer present, the patient is committed to taking the medication for life. It is important, however, to be aware of medications that produce dependancy; when these medications are to be discontinued, they should not be stopped abruptly, but reduced slowly over time so that discontinuation can be accomplished without undue discomfort. This is especially important when opioid-dependent individuals require admission to the hospital for treatment of an acute illness, because discontinuation of the routine regimen for pain relief, which is all too frequently done, may lead to withdrawal and unnecessary complications in the management of the presenting illness.

*Tolerance* is a feature of all opioid medications. The medication becomes less effective with time. Tolerance both to the beneficial and to the adverse effects of the medication can develop. Tolerance to the psychological benefits of a substance is also seen in addiction and is one of the phenomena that underlies the escalation of dose in substance use. When tolerance develops in the normal course of opioid therapy, individuals frequently complain of increased levels of pain or that the medication does not work for as long a period as it had originally. When tolerance develops, pain relief usually can be re-established by increasing the dose of medication. However, dose adjustments must be made in consultation with the prescribing physician whose determination of dosing change is based on a consideration of the potential for changes in the underlying medical condition (recurrence of a cancer, worsening of arthritis), changes in the treatment of coexisting problems (addition of a conflicting medication), and the development of adverse effects that may have resulted in a reduction in pain control. In general, when an appropriate dose of medication is determined, tolerance develops gradually. It is important to realize that, in individuals who have developed tolerance to medications, the doses of opioid analgesics that would normally control pain or anesthetics that would normally produce surgical levels of sedation and analgesia in a nontolerant individual are likely to be ineffective in managing pain. This becomes important when someone who requires a regular dosing of opioid medication to maintain pain control requires a surgical procedure. Higher doses must be given to achieve the desired level of control both for surgical anesthesia and postoperative pain control.

Finally, *pseudoaddiction* is a condition in which individuals seek additional medications for an inadequately treated pain condition. Such individuals frequent emergency rooms and visit multiple physicians in a quest to find relief from their pain. The behavior often is viewed as being associated with the drug-seeking behavior of a drug addict. If an effective treatment is identified and an adequate amount of medication is provided, the drug-seeking behavior for these individuals is no longer a problem. Unfortunately, pseudoaddiction is under-recognized when it involves opioid medications, although similar behavior could be seen in cases in which insufficient dosing of nitroglycerin were given for the treatment of chest pain or if an inadequate insulin supply was provided to manage diabetes.

## WILL USE OF THESE MEDICATIONS SHORTEN MY LIFE?

This questions is usually posed from one of two perspectives. The first perspective is that of someone who has had a relative or loved one who took opioid medications to manage pain during and, especially, at the end of a terminal disease, and thereafter succumbed to the disease within a relatively short period of time after starting opioid treatment. The other perspective often is based on television, movie, or media depictions of someone who has been addicted to a similar medication and is in poor health, or someone who had experienced an unpleasant or violent end to their life reportedly in association with the use of an opioid medication. Much of the information about long-term or regular use of opioid medications has come from these two populations. In fact, short life expectancies following the initiation of opioid pain control has been the rule only because, until recently, opioids have been deemed only appropriate to manage the pain of terminal disease, such as cancer and AIDS, that have a limited survival. The patients, however, generally succumb to the disease, rather that to the pain medications provided. The likelihood that life expectancy would be shortened by the regular use of an opioid medication alone is no more likely than for any other prescription medication taken appropriately for the management of a life-altering condition. It might further be argued that a life of uncontrolled pain is likely to be shorter and certainly less pleasant than a life in which the pain is properly managed with opioid medications. The adverse effects of uncontrolled pain frequently are not considered, but include increased stress that can lead to a decreased immune response with a concomitant increased risk of infection and some cancers, an increase in gastrointestinal complications such as ulcers, and an increase in blood pressure with the accompanying increased risk of heart attack and stroke. Therefore, the complications of uncontrolled pain alone may result in a shortened life expectancy.

## WILL THE MEDICATIONS LOSE THEIR EFFECT TO THE POINT WHERE THEY WILL NO LONGER CONTROL PAIN?

The answer to this concern can serve to answer similar objections to the prescribing of opioid medications that are posed by both health care and legal systems: *Should there be a limit to the number of pills prescribed to treat any pain problem?* The direct answer to the question is that a particular dose of a medication may lose its effect, but it is usually possible to achieve adequate pain control by increasing the dose of medication as tolerance develops or as the basic pain condition changes. As noted earlier in this chapter, one of the characteristic features of opioid medications is the development of tolerance to both the adverse and beneficial effects of the medication. This is both a blessing and a curse when attempting to achieve adequate pain control using an opioid medication. The fact that many of the adverse effects of the medications disappear or diminish significantly with time makes it possible to eventually achieve good pain control with minimal adverse effects, although this process may be slow. Unfortunately, with time, tolerance can develop to the beneficial effects of the medication, thus necessitating an increase in the amount of drug required to produce adequate pain control. Slow increases in opioid dosing can be made indefinitely and will continue to produce increases in pain relief, because many opioid medications do not have a ceiling dose above which no further pain relief can be achieved. The ultimate dosing limit is therefore not determined by a predetermined dose, but rather by therapeutic benefit—a balance between optimum pain control and the development of adverse effects for an individual pain sufferer. The dose per milligram of drug necessary to control any individual's pain is determined by the effectiveness of the drug to control the pain for that individual and the individual's ability to tolerate a particular dose of the medication. The number of pills required to deliver the appropriate number of milligrams of drug for adequate pain relief is determined by amount of drug a manufacturer places in each of the pills. For example, if 100 mg of a given drug is required to control pain for 1 day, one would need to take more 5-mg pills (20/day) to control the pain than if 50-mg pills (two/day) are prescribed. This logic seems intuitive, however, administrative decisions and punitive allegations are not infrequently based on the number of pills given rather than the milligrams required. Therefore, the proper dosing of medication should be based on good clinical judgment that is the result of careful comprehensive evaluation and determination of tolerability and response for each individual.

# CHAPTER 9

# Pharmacologic Options in Pain Management— Adjuvant Medications

Until recently, the nonopioid and opioid analgesic medications have been the first and often only medications considered for the management of pain. This approach to pain management has led to frustration on the part the of pain sufferer, who frequently complains that his pain is inadequately managed, and on the part of the physician, who believes all known treatment options have been exhausted. Fortunately, over the last several years, through closer communication between clinicians and basic scientists, many of the observations made in basic-science research laboratories are being applied in clinical practice. By coupling the knowledge of how different drugs work to produce their desired effect with the knowledge of how pain is perceived and processed, it was hypothesized that certain drugs designed for purposes other than to treat pain—such as those used to treat depression, seizures, or blood pressure—might indeed affect the pain pathway and thus aid in relieving pain. The addition of these so called *adjuvant medications* to previously recognized treatment regimens for pain has significantly improved our ability to control pain. Indeed, adjuvant medications have been found to produce better pain relief than typical analgesics when used in the management of neuropathic pain.

Adjuvant medications are numerous and may be found listed among several different drug classifications. Although certain medications seem to be used more than others as first-choice medications for managing pain, none of the alternatives is beneficial in all situations, and none seems to be significantly better than another with respect to pain relief.

The selection of adjuvant medications is based at least as often on safety, ease of dosing, cost, and potentially beneficial adverse effects, such as drowsiness for those with insomnia and weight loss for those who are overweight, than on actual pain-relieving potential. Initial selections that fail to relieve pain often are abandoned for the next alternative with a not surprisingly diminishing likelihood for success with each subsequent selection.

Because adjuvant medications cross pharmacologic boundaries for practicing specialties, a reluctance frequently exists on the part of the prescribing physician to utilize certain adjuvant medications to their potential, due to a lack of familiarity or comfort with medications not typically used within their particular area of practice. Unfortunately, inadequate dosing often leads to the perception that the medication provided is not beneficial; this may result in discontinuation of a useful medication and lack of its further consideration in subsequent treatment. It is therefore important to keep a record of all medications that have been tried to alleviate pain, the highest doses used, and the reason for discontinuation.

In most instances, it is preferable to treat a particular medical problem with a single medication. This practice makes it easier to determine whether or not the medication being used is beneficial, and whether it is responsible for producing adverse effects if they occur. Because the perception of pain relies on many different biologic processes, however, it is unlikely that a single medication, working through a single mechanism, will suffice in eliminating the noxious signal. Therefore, pain is often more effectively treated when low doses of several medications with different mechanisms of action are used in concert, rather than large doses of a single medication. A compromise between the two approaches is to start one medication at a time to determine its contribution to pain control and add medications with different mechanisms of action in an attempt to intervene in as many places as necessary to produce relief. The broad spectrum of adjuvant medications offers a wide variety of mechanisms of action that may influence the pain pathway in many different ways. Alternate medications with different mechanisms of action usually are added to an existing regimen that is tolerated, but only partially effective, in the hope of eliminating pain. If pain is eventually controlled, a process of reducing the doses of one medication at a time is tried to determine the lowest dose of each medication necessary to maintain pain control. Thus, the variety of treatment plans reflects a careful orchestration between the different drug mechanisms, tailored to the specific pain sufferer's ability to respond to and tolerate the combinations.

## ANTICONVULSANTS

The best known and most frequently used adjuvant medications are the anticonvulsants (Table 9-1) used for treating seizures. In current practice, the anticonvulsant medications are used preferentially, because intolerable adverse effects seem to occur less frequently with their use. For years, the anticonvulsant medication carbamazepine (Tegretol) was the first choice for treating neuropathic pain related to trigeminal neuralgia. It was initially considered as a treatment option because the pres-

**Table 9-1** Anticonvulsant Medications Used in Pain Management

| Drug | Dose Range | Adverse Effects |
|---|---|---|
| Gabapentin (Neurontin®) | 200-3600 mg/day | Drowsiness, dizziness |
| Oxcarbazepine (Trileptal®) | 150-1800 mg/day | Drowsiness, lightheadedness, dizziness |
| Levetiracetam (Keppra®) | 250-1500 mg/day | Drowsiness, dizziness |
| Topiramate (Topamax®) | 100-400 mg/day | Drowsiness, cognitive suppression |
| Lamotrigine (Lamictal®) | 50-200 mg/day | Rash, fatigue, stomach upset |
| Carbamazepine (Tegretol®) | 100-1600 mg/day | Drowsiness, bone marrow suppression, kidney stones |
| Zonisamide (Zonegran®) | 100-600 mg/day | Drowsiness, weight loss, dizziness |
| Pregabalin (Lyrica®) | 150-600 mg/day | Drowsiness, dizziness |
| Tiagabine (Gabatril®) | 4-16 mg/day | Dizziness, lightheadedness, fatigue |
| Phenytoin (Dilantin®) | 200-600 mg/day | Double vision, imbalance, slurred speech |
| Clonazepam (Klonopin®) | 2-7 mg/day | Drowsiness, disequilibrium, abnormal behavior |

entation and course of facial pain associated with trigeminal neuralgia seemed similar to that of a seizure. It was found to be effective for this problem and other neuropathic conditions such as shingles and sciatica. Although carbamazepine produced less drowsiness and memory problems than does phenytoin (Dilantin, another anticonvulsant in frequent use), there remained a rare, but serious adverse effect associated with its use: It could prevent the production of blood cells. Carbamazepine also affected its own detoxification in the liver, as well as the detoxification of other medications. This feature of the drug contributed further to problems related to its use.

With the introduction of newer anticonvulsants that are easier to use with fewer serious side effects, a dramatic shift has occurred toward their use in pain management. The first of these newer medications was *gabapentin* (Neurontin). Gabapentin was initially designed to work in a fashion similar to the major brain chemical responsible for reducing nerve cell activity, gamma-aminobutyric acid (GABA). Unlike the older anticonvulsants, gabapentin did not influence liver or kidney function, did not interact with other medications, and had very few significant adverse effects. Gabapentin was found to be at least as effective as carbamazepine for most individuals, and was especially effective in reducing the burning quality of neuropathic pain. It was well tolerated by most individuals, who typically experienced only mild lightheadedness and drowsiness as the most frequent adverse effects. Some individuals noted weight gain. Because gabapentin proved so successful for improving pain control for previously unmanageable pain, other anticonvulsant medications were tried when pain was inadequately controlled with gabapentin. The anticonvulsant medications in current use are listed Table 9-1, with features that tend to influence where they rank in the selection sequence as treatment options. It should be noted, although many of these medications frequently are prescribed to improve pain control, most of the medications have not been approved by the Food and Drug Administration (FDA) for use in the treatment of pain, and they have yet to undergo the scrutiny of controlled clinical trials to substantiate their role in pain management.

## ANTIDEPRESSANTS

The other group of adjuvant medications considered as first-line treatment options are the tricyclic antidepressants (Table 9-2). These medications, represented by amitriptyline (Elavil), nortriptyline (Pamelor), desipramine (Norpramin), doxepin (Sinequan), and imipramine (Tofranil), influence the activity of many chemicals in the brain that reduce nerve cell firing. Of these medications, amitriptyline has been studied most extensively and is still considered high on the list of medications selected for treating neuropathic pain. Unfortunately, the tricyclic antidepressants influence many systems other than those involved in the pain pathway and therefore are plagued by numerous broad-ranging adverse effects. The adverse effects include dry mouth, constipation, drowsiness, weight gain, low blood pressure, rapid heart beat, urinary retention, dizziness, blurring of vision, aggravation of glaucoma, and an increased risk of seizures. These medications must therefore be used with caution in individuals who are overweight, have a seizure disorder, or have underlying heart problems; they are used frequently for those pain sufferers with coexisting insomnia. The pain control achieved with the tricyclic antidepressants appears to be related to the many mechanisms through which they influence the pain pathway, because newer antidepressants that work through very selective mechanisms of action, such as fluoxetine (Prozac), sertraline (Zoloft), paroxetine (Paxil), escitalopram (Lexapro), and citalopram (Celexa), seem to produce little benefit with respect to pain control unless an underlying primary depression or psychogenic condition is present to potentiate the pain problem. In those cases, significant pain relief may be realized.

Other antidepressants, including venlafaxine, bupropion, trazodone, and mirtazapine, whose mechanisms of action and side effect profiles lie somewhere between the two extremes, have been used with varying degrees of success due more to the improved side-effect profile than to pain control. The newest of this group of medications, *duloxetine* (Cymbalta), which has indications for use both for depression and for neuropathic pain, offers an additional option for adjuvant care. Its role in pain management is promising, but is yet to be evaluated.

**Table 9-2** Antidepressant Medications Used in Pain Management

| Drug | Dose Range | Adverse Effects |
|------|-----------|-----------------|
| Amitriptyline (Elavil®) | 10-150 mg/day | Drowsiness, dry mouth, weight gain, constipation, seizures, cardiac toxicity, urinary retention |
| Nortriptyline (Pamelor®) | 10-150 mg/day | Drowsiness, dry mouth, weight gain, constipation, seizures, cardiac toxicity, urinary retention |
| Doxepin (Sinequan®) | 25-150 mg/day | Drowsiness, dry mouth, weight gain, constipation, seizures, cardiac toxicity, urinary retention |
| Imipramine (Tofranil®) | 25-200 mg/day | Drowsiness, dry mouth, weight gain, constipation, seizures, cardiac toxicity, urinary retention |
| Desipramine (Norpramin®) | 50-200 mg/day | Drowsiness, dry mouth, weight gain, constipation, seizures, cardiac toxicity, urinary retention |
| Duloxitine (Cymbalta®) | 30-120 mg/day | Insomnia, nausea, dizziness, fatigue, constipation |
| Venlafaxin (Effexor®) | 37.5-225 mg/day | High blood pressure, weight loss, dry mouth, impotence, tremor |
| Bupropion (Wellbutrin®) | 75-225 mg/day | Anorexia, headache, dry mouth, agitation, tremor |
| Trazadone (Desyrel®) | 50-400 mg/day | Drowsiness, nausea, vomiting, priapism |
| Mirtazapine (Remeron®) | 20-50 mg/day | Drowsiness, weight gain, dizziness, dry mouth |
| Fluoxitine (Prozac®) | 5-60 mg/day | Anxiety, nervousness, insomnia, tremor, chest pain, diarrhea |
| Paroxetine (Paxil®) | 20-50 mg/day | Drowsiness, dizziness, insomnia, headache |
| Sertraline (Zoloft®) | 50-200 mg/day | Nausea, insomnia, diarrhea, dry mouth, tremor |
| Escitalopram (Lexapro®) | 10-20 mg/day | Nausea, insomnia, fatigue, drowsiness |
| Citalopram (Celexa®) | 20-40 mg/day | Dry mouth, sweating, nausea, insomnia, tremor, agitation, diarrhea |

## ANTISPASMODIC AGENTS

*Baclofen* (Lioresal), an antispasmodic agent (Table 9-3), is the second-line treatment for trigeminal neuralgia following, and often in combination with, carbamazepine. This medication works in a fashion similar to GABA in the spinal cord and thereby reduces the likelihood that a pain signal would be transmitted beyond its entry into the nervous system. Baclofen produces mild pain relief in some individuals, but may cause drowsiness, lightheadedness, nausea, and vomiting. One caution with the use of baclofen is that it should be discontinued slowly if it has been taken for more than 2 months, because sudden discontinuation may result in hallucinations, seizures, or both.

*Tizanidine* (Zanaflex) is a medication intended for the treatment of the spasticity associated with cerebral palsy and multiple sclerosis. It works in a fashion similar to the blood pressure medication clonidine, but has less influence on heart and blood vessels. Because of the central site of action, individuals taking tizanidine typically experience less lightheadedness on rising from a supine to a sitting or from a sitting to a standing position than if they were taking clonidine. Tizanidine produces its analgesic effect by decreasing the amount of pain-signal transmission through the zone of entry to higher levels of the central nervous system (Figure 4-5). Tizanidine has been used with some success in

**Table 9-3** Antispasmodic Medications Used in Pain Management

| Drug | Dose Range | Adverse Effects |
|---|---|---|
| Tizanidine (Zanaflex®) | 2-52 mg/day | Drowsiness, lightheadedness, low blood pressure |
| Baclofen (Lioresal®) | 50-80 mg/day | Drowsiness, lightheadedness, dizziness |
| Cyclobenzaprine (Flexeril®) | 15-30 mg/day | Drowsiness, dry mouth, dizziness, fatigue, confusion |
| Methocarbamol (Robaxin®) | 1500-4000 mg/day | Headache, fever, low blood pressure, slow heart rate |
| Carisoprodol (Soma®) | 350-1400 mg/day | Drowsiness, dizziness, irritability, headache, rapid heart rate, abuse potential |

the treatment of pain related to multifocal muscle spasm, and it has produced some mild reduction in neuropathic pain. Its most frequent adverse effect is drowsiness. It is typically dosed at bedtime, and most individuals report less of a "hangover" effect with tizanidine than is experienced with the tricyclic antidepressants. The drowsiness experienced often precludes the dosing of tizanidine during waking hours.

Other antispasmodic agents, including cyclobenzaprine, methocarbamol, and carisoprodol, that have been used to treat pain associated with muscle spasm have not played a role in the treatment of neuropathic pain.

## MISCELLANEOUS AGENTS

A number of other medications (Table 9-4) have been used with mixed success in the treatment of pain. *Clonidine* (Catapres) is an antihypertensive medication that, through its central action, has the potential for reducing neuropathic pain. However, due to its significant peripheral effect, it can produce undesirable lightheadedness and drowsiness. These adverse effects are most profound when the medication is taken by mouth, which requires circulation throughout the body and delivery of relatively small amounts of medication to the desired site. Clonidine, however, also is available in a patch formulation that delivers the med-

**Table 9-4** Miscellaneous Agents Used in Pain Management

| Drug | Dose Range | Adverse Effects |
|---|---|---|
| Mexiletine (Mexitil®) | 150-1800 mg/day | Abnormal heart rates and rhythm, nausea, tremor, confusion |
| Clonidine (Catapres-TTS®) | 0.1-0.3 mg/day | Drowsiness, dry mouth, constipation, low blood pressure |
| Capsaicin (Zostrix®, Axsain®) | 0.025-0.075% 3-4 times/day | Burning, skin irritation |
| Lidocaine 5% (Lidoderm®) | 1-4 patches 12 hours/day | Skin irritation |
| Custom formulated compounds | 3-4 times/day | Skin irritation |

ication through the skin and then ultimately throughout the body. If the patch is placed over or near an area of superficial neuropathic pain, the resulting concentration of medication is highest in the area where it can have its greatest effect and less in other regions of the body. In painful localized conditions, such as those associated with an eruption of shingles after the vesicles have healed (postherpetic neuralgia), locally applied clonidine can decrease the release of chemicals from nerve terminals in the skin that would otherwise increase the likelihood that a pain signal would be generated; thus, the analgesic effect may be realized at doses that do not produce significant adverse effects.

Local anesthetic medications are typically thought of when pain from a surgical procedure, such as that experienced during the drilling of a dental cavity or the suturing of a deep cut in the skin, is to be prevented. Local anesthetics, when applied in more unusual ways, however, also may be effective as adjuvant treatment for neuropathic pain, although technically the effect is more precisely that of a nonopioid analgesic administered systemically, rather than as an adjuvant. Two formulations of note in this regard are mexiletine and lidocaine. *Mexiletine* (Mexitil) is an orally administered local anesthetic agent that is more often used in the treatment of abnormalities in heart rhythm. In this role, mexiletine blocks the conduction of abnormal impulses that, when generated in the heart, result in inappropriate heart beats and inefficient pumping of blood to the lungs and throughout the body. The same mechanism that blocks the abnormal impulses blocks the transmission of pain signals in peripheral nerve cells, thereby decreasing the amount of pain perceived. Although potentially beneficial, mexiletine can unfortunately produce abnormal heart rhythms by blocking the normal impulses generated in the heart for coordinating the regular heart beat.

In addition to its more traditional injectable formulation, *lidocaine* has recently become available in a patch formulation (Lidoderm) that may be applied topically to painful areas for relief. As with other topically applied preparations, the medication has minimal influence on body functions distant to the site of application; therefore, it produces few general adverse effects. The lidocaine patch is most effective for the control of superficial pain, such as that associated with postherpetic neuralgia, but pain control in deeper structures may be achieved with regular use. The patches may be applied for periods of 12 hours, but should be removed for 12 hours between doses to prevent nerve damage that can occur with prolonged exposure of nerve to local anesthetic agents. The most frequent complication related to the use of the lidocaine patch is a local skin reaction associated with the adhesive used to make the patch adhere to the skin. Irritation associated with repeated patch application and removal can be reduced by varying the location of the patch.

# CHAPTER 10

# Pharmacologic Options in Pain Management— Dosing and Alternate Routes of Administration

W HEN PRESCRIBING MEDICATION for adequate pain relief, the challenge for the health care professional is to establish a level of medication for the individual suffering pain in such a way that optimum pain relief is achieved without adverse effects. When the optimum medication level is attained, the dosing is said to be in the *therapeutic range*. For any given medication, a dose exists below which benefit is not achieved (*subtherapeutic range*) and above which adverse effects occur (*toxic range*). The amount of medication given should be sufficient to produce pain relief without adverse effects, and should be given frequently enough to prevent the pain from returning prior to the next scheduled dose. In practice, it may not be possible to eliminate pain completely. In that case, the best result is to maintain pain levels within a tolerable range without adverse effects. An ideal delivery system would provide, through constant monitoring, just the right amount of medication necessary, only when the need arises. This would be similar to the minute-to-minute adjustment of heart rate and breathing during cycles of rest and exertion. This level of control over medication delivery is generally too cumbersome and costly for general use. In the best of situations, the therapeutic range may be achieved with once-a-day pulse dosing or with a reservoir of medication that is released steadily over a period of days.

Unfortunately, as illustrated in Figure 10-1, when higher doses of medication are required, toxic effects may occur. Lower doses must then

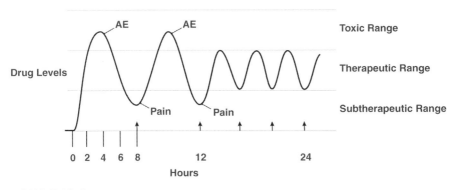

**FIGURE 10-1**

Rationale for selecting dosing strengths and intervals. Doses should be sufficient to control pain (therapeutic range), but low enough to avoid adverse
effects (AE; toxic range). Dosing should be frequent enough to avoid drug
levels that are insufficient for pain control (subtherapeutic range).
(Modified from Figure 51.7 in *Textbook of Pain*, Fourth Edition by Patrick D.
Wall and Ronald Melzack, 1999. Reprinted with permission from Elsevier.)

be given more often to prevent pain from returning. To maintain uniform pain relief around the clock, immediate-release formulations must
be given frequently, approximately every 4 to 6 hours. To achieve the
greatest pain relief with fewest adverse effects, the dosing should be
given regularly and on the clock; that is, a dose prescribed every 6 hours
should be take at 6 AM, 12 PM, 6 PM, and 12 AM, rather than four times
during the waking hours. Frequent dosing regimens, however, are difficult for most people to follow. Doses often are delayed or forgotten, and
nighttime doses interrupt sleep. For this reason, sustained-release preparations are preferred for maintenance dosing regimens. Morphine is
available in preparations that release the drug over either a 12- or 24-
hour period, thereby reducing the need for frequent dosing.

Using pulsed dosing, many methods of delivery may be used to
achieve a stable blood level of medication. By far the easiest and most
frequently used route of administration is the oral route. Oral-delivery
drugs typically are available in liquid, tablet, or capsule form. The rate of
medication delivery is determined by the properties of the delivery system and the state of the gut. Medications are swallowed, released from
the delivery source, and then absorbed by various, and often limited,

portions of the intestinal lining. It is important that medication be released from the source when it is in that portion of the intestine that can absorb it, otherwise adequate medication will not be delivered. If the intestinal contents are moving too quickly, and medication is released too slowly, potentially available medication may pass the sites of absorption. This would be analogous to driving too fast on the highway and not being able to use a desired exit ramp. Conversely, although rare, slowed intestinal transit times may result in absorption of greater than expected amounts of drug, thus leading to toxicity. In general, extended- or controlled-release systems are designed to deliver a predetermined amount of medication over a prolonged period to reduce the need for frequent dosing.

These formulations should not be modified before they are taken. Crushing pills or breaking open capsules of controlled-delivery systems negates the carefully engineered delivery system and leads to a rapid release of larger amounts of medication than intended. This may lead to serious toxic adverse effects. Crushing or splitting pills is generally not a problem with preparations that are designed for immediate release.

All components of medications (pill coatings, drug, and fillers) are controlled and tested to give reproducible medication delivery. Variations in the effectiveness of generic formulations when compared with brand preparations usually are related to differences in the delivery system, pill coats, and fillers, rather than to the drug being dispensed. Although differences in response to treatment with brand name and generic medications generally do not occur, it may be important to consider the variation in generic preparations prior to discontinuing a potentially effective medication because of an inconsistent response.

The oral route of drug administration may be influenced by diet and the general medical condition of the individual taking the medication. Although many medications, especially the anti-inflammatory agents, are better tolerated when taken with food, it is important to be aware that intestinal contents may influence medication delivery. Some foods may reduce the rate of absorption, whereas others may enhance it. Certain foods, like grapefruit, also may affect drug metabolism by influencing enzymes in the body that eliminate certain drugs. It is therefore important to consider and address potential dietary interactions before beginning an oral drug regimen.

Unfortunately, in conditions such as gastrointestinal cancer and degenerative diseases of the nervous system, swallowing is not possible. In cases of severe acute pain, such as that associated with migraine headache or an attack of acute appendicitis, the body's ability to absorb medications taken by mouth from the intestinal track is reduced. In these cases, medications still may be delivered via components of the gastrointestinal system. Atomized sprays are readily absorbed through the nasal mucosa and oral pharynx, some medications are formulated in tablets designed to dissolve under the tongue and be absorbed through the lining of the oral cavity, and suppository formulations deliver medication to the lining of the rectum, where they may be absorbed. The rectal route of administration tends to be least favored by many individuals, yet it is important to know that therapeutic doses of medication may be delivered in this fashion. Many analgesic medications not routinely available in suppository form can be specially prepared by a pharmacist to deliver the required medication.

When the gastrointestinal system cannot be utilized for drug delivery, alternate routes of drug administration must be considered if pain relief is to be achieved. In the hospital setting, medications often are given by injection beneath the skin, into muscle, into veins or arteries, or into a body cavity. *Intravenous injection* produces the most rapid response, but care must be taken not to produce significant toxic effects, because maximum blood levels for each dose are achieved at the end of the injection. Dosing can be adjusted to need, but this may be labor intensive and less than optimum in some busy hospital settings. In an attempt to improve adequate pain management in the hospital setting, the technology for intravenous infusion has advanced to provide an infusion of medication through a mechanical pump. The technology is called *patient-controlled analgesia* or PCA. In the design of the PCA pump, it is recognized that a constant infusion of a particular dose of medication may be insufficient to manage pain around the clock, because pain varies throughout a 24-hour period due to an individual's level of personal or disease activity. Thus, in addition to a predetermined regular rate of delivery, a quantity of medication is available on-demand by pressing a button when needed. The amount of each on-demand dosing and the number of doses allowed is predetermined and limited by a "lock out" command to reduce the possibility of overmedication. The number of on-demand doses and the response to treatment then is monitored over a 24-hour period to determine the amount of medication required to control pain. The rate of continuous infusion then is adjusted in an attempt to decrease the need for on-demand dosing. PCA administration of medication usually results in overall lower medication utilization and greater patient satisfaction related to their pain control.

Drug levels reach their maximum more slowly with *other forms of injection* and usually are administered at intervals rather than continuously. The rate at which drug enters the circulation depends on the available blood supply serving the area of injection, the surface area available for contact with blood vessels, and the fluid or vehicle in which the drug is suspended. In general, medication is absorbed most rapidly from the lining of the body cavity, next from muscle, and least from within the skin. Further modification of the rate of absorption often is accomplished by the concomitant administration of a drug like epinephrine, which decreases the diameter of blood vessels and reduces blood flow that would otherwise increase the absorption and decrease the duration of effect through drug clearance. Medications are absorbed more quickly from water- or saline-based preparations than from oil-based suspensions. Although relatively safe and generally well tolerated (with the exception of the needle stick), the insertion of a needle into areas of the body that cannot be visualized may result in inadvertent damage to deep-lying blood vessels or nerves—this can be uncomfortable for the one on the sharp end of the needle. Frequent dosing increases the risk of complications.

For those not in a hospital setting, the most frequently used alternative to the gastrointestinal track for drug administration is the *topical* or *transdermal route* of administration. Topical preparations are available as commercially produced or specially compounded creams, gels, lotions, or patches that are applied to the skin. The beneficial effect of creams, gels, and lotion compounds is of short duration, but even short-term relief can be helpful in localized areas for individuals who cannot tolerate the medications when delivered via other routes. Transdermal patches provide more prolonged relief through varied systems. Patches are generally constructed of a flexible material, within which is enclosed a reservoir of medication and a filter system designed to release a controlled rate of medication. The delivery system is applied to an area of non-hairy skin and held in place by adhesive. The time during which medication is continuously released varies from 8 hours to 1 week. The greatest benefit achieved by using transdermal systems is that uniform medication delivery can be achieved over an extended period. The infrequency with which patches require changing frees the pain sufferer from needing to return regularly to the medicine bottle for relief. With the addition of a new PCA technology (Ionsys) that drives medication on-demand through the skin using a low-level electrical current (*iontophoretic delivery*), breakthrough dosing (medication needed for intermittent episodes of pain that exceeds the coverage provided by the routine, scheduled dosing regimen) also should be available through transdermal administration. Iontophoretic delivery has the advantage of not needing the preparation of an intravenous access site.

Finally, when intolerable adverse effects occur in the absence of adequate pain relief, medications may be delivered directly to the brain and spinal cord, where the receptors responsible for much of the pain relief are located. This method of delivery, called *intrathecal infusion*, provides more medication closer to the site where it produces its effect and less medication to body regions where the effects are unwanted. Intrathecal infusion is used infrequently because of the degree of invasiveness of the procedures necessary to provide the mechanism of delivery. Intrathecal infusion requires the placement of a tube inside the vertebral canal and into the membrane-covered reservoir of spinal fluid (the *thecal sac*) that contains and protects the spinal cord and nerve roots. A surgical procedure then is necessary to anchor the tube and implant a medication reservoir and pumping system under the skin. The benefit of this route of administration is that a steady dose of medication is delivered to potentially provide for improved, uniform pain control and fewer general adverse effects. The limitations of the technique include a relatively high incidence of failure, the need for a surgical procedure to implant a pumping system for drug delivery, and the potential for pump malfunctions and surgical complications. At present, few approved options are available for alternative infusible medications if adverse effects occur or tolerance develops. The medications most frequently delivered by this method are morphine (for pain) and baclofen (primarily for spasticity). Other medications less frequently used in intrathecal pumps include bupivacaine, hydromorphone, clonidine, physostigmine, and ketamine. Ziconotide (Prialt) is the newest of the intrathecally administered medications to gain approval for pain relief. This potentially promising drug is derived from the toxin of a species of cone snail indigenous to the waters of the Pacific Ocean. Ziconotide has been found to be beneficial for the treatment of both nociceptive and neuropathic pain. It is not an opioid medication, so unlike morphine, tolerance and physical dependency do not develop with ziconotide. Its primary limitation is that a very narrow dosing range is available in which pain relief can be achieved without causing adverse effects. These adverse effects can include nausea, confusion, agitation, blurring of vision, headache, drowsiness, and urinary retention. Failure of this method of medication delivery is significantly reduced with careful screening prior to pump placement. However, even in the best outcomes, individuals may require some oral medications to achieve adequate pain control.

Many routes of administration are at the disposal of the health care provider to aid in delivering the best analgesic care possible. In general, the choice of route of administration is made on the basis of the type of pain to be treated, what is most convenient, and what is least invasive. A knowledge of all alternatives is necessary to make it possible to choose the most appropriate route for the individual requiring care.

# CHAPTER 11

# Invasive Options and When to Consider Them

ALTHOUGH CONSERVATIVE, noninvasive management of chronic pain is preferred, instances occur in which more aggressive means of treatment are necessary. As with medication options, a spectrum of invasive options is available to improve a chronic pain condition. These options range from minimally invasive to extensive operative reconstruction. It is important to realize that many conditions that produce chronic pain will resolve in time, using conservative management, and that many procedures, in the process of correcting an obvious problem, produce irreversible changes that must be dealt with for the remainder of an individual's life. It is important to know when and why an invasive treatment is best.

Several reasons exist to consider an invasive procedure. The first reason is clear. Because pain alerts an individual to the presence of actual or potential tissue injury, responses directed toward correction of the cause of the pain may preserve life and function, while relieving pain. Invasive procedures often are necessary to preserve life in emergency situations. Examples of this include establishing an airway for someone who has aspirated a foreign object when a Heimlich maneuver has been ineffective, or providing emergent care for stabilization of someone who has been injured as a result of a serious motor vehicle accident. Invasive procedures also are essential when employed to correct conditions such as compression of the spinal cord, nerve roots, or blood vessels by a protruding intervertebral disk, an invading cancer, or a foreign object that, if left untreated, would lead to paralysis or loss of function. They also are necessary to prevent further complications from acute medical conditions such as appendicitis. Many of the procedures used either restore or approximate the structural integrity of an injured organ and aid in healing; others can affect a cure.

A second reason to consider an invasive procedure is to provide or refine a diagnosis when noninvasive means have been insufficient to reveal the source of pain. Such procedures improve planning and appropriately define and focus efforts for ultimate treatment. Contrast (dye)-assisted radiographs (x-ray), computerized tomography (CT) scans, or magnetic resonance imaging (MRI) are used to locate and define the size of tumors in individuals with cancer, the extent of blood vessel blockade in people with heart disease, and the presence of nerve root compression associated with a bulging intervertebral disk. The precise injection of anesthetic agents that block the conduction of nerve impulses also are used to identify and confirm which nerves are responsible for a persistent pain signal.

A third reason for performing invasive procedures is to provide comfort in terminal disease. Large cancerous tumors can compress or invade adjacent nerves, blood vessels, and organs, which can lead to compromised functioning and discomfort. Procedures that reduce the tumor mass can reduce pain through decompression of sensitive structures. Cutting portions of the pain pathways can eliminate regional pain by preventing the effective transmission of the pain signal to the thalamus, the portion of the brain where pain is consciously perceived. The medical status of the individual, the prognosis for survival, and the potential for improved quality of life following recovery from the procedure are essential factors that determine whether a procedure should be considered and what type of procedure should be done.

Invasive procedures also should be considered when conservative management has failed to achieve the desired recovery, and effective, invasive intervention is available. Invasive procedures for pain control are evolving, but to date, no clear panacea for all conditions has emerged. Unfortunately, if applied to the wrong individual or wrong condition, it is not uncommon to experience a permanent worsening of the pain or the creation of a new uncomfortable condition. The resulting pain is often less manageable than the original pain. The success of invasive procedures depends greatly on the careful screening and selection of individuals for whom a procedure is being contemplated. It is important to identify both those likely to benefit and those for whom the procedure is likely to fail. Many factors play a role in determining the likelihood of a favorable outcome: general medical condition, drug and smoking history, and nontangible factors that include psychosocial, employment, and litigation status. The use of invasive procedures for pain control should be carefully considered.

The invasive procedures available for managing chronic pain range from the minimally invasive, in which the intervention is administered through a needle or instrument port (a small incision for inserting a viewing camera and cable-controlled instruments), to the fully open operative procedures. The advantages of the minimally invasive procedures are that they can frequently be accomplished in an office setting or in a same-day surgical unit, usually require minimal anesthetic support, have a relatively low incidence of complication, and are generally less costly than major operations. In contrast, major operations more often require general anesthesia, more frequently leave permanent scars, require periods of postoperative observation and recovery, and have longer periods of recovery, all of which contributes to overall cost.

*Minimally invasive procedures* most often are employed for the purposes of managing acute pain, acute exacerbations of chronic pain, and for establishing a diagnosis. *Nerve blocks* involve the injection or infiltration of a local anesthetic agent, such as lidocaine or bupivacaine, in tissue closely associated with a nerve. Most individuals have experienced this procedure at the dentist's office, when an injection is provided to eliminate the pain expected when a tooth is drilled. The same procedure may be used to produce pain relief in regions supplied by any nerve that can be reached with a needle, whether to reduce discomfort related to a procedure or to a recurrent spontaneous pain. Depending on the desired outcome, the medications delivered can vary. Frequently, steroids are added to the local anesthetic injection to provide relief from any inflammatory process present at the site of the injection. The name given to the specific block usually denotes the nerve or site of injection (occipital nerve block, ulnar nerve block), the route taken by the needle (the *caudal block* for gynecological anesthesia enters the spinal canal at the base of the spine), or the medication delivered (a combination of a long-acting steroid and a local anesthetic usually is administered in an *epidural steroid injection*). Similar techniques are used to provide medication to individual joint spaces such as the shoulder, sacroiliac, hip, knee joints, and the joints between the bones of the vertebral column. When effective, injections of local anesthetic agents and steroids provide temporary relief for acute pain or pain exacerbations ranging from several hours to several weeks in some cases. However, the utility of these injections for the management of chronic pain conditions is poor. Frequent injections increase the risk of complications related to the needle insertion, such as deep lacerations, bleeding, and nerve injury, as well as complications associated with chronic steroid use.

Regional anesthesia also may be provided for an entire limb by delivering the anesthetic drug into the venous system after temporarily blocking of the flow of blood with a tourniquet for 5 to 10 minutes. This procedure is less invasive than those involving deep needle insertions. It is most frequently used in the diagnosis of limb-based neuropathic pain that is presumed to be maintained through activity of the sympathetic nervous system. For this procedure, drugs that block the effect of the sympathetic nervous system are injected into the vein of a limb whose circulation has been isolated from the rest of the body by a tourniquet, to determine whether pain can be reduced. Possible complications of this procedure include nerve injury due to prolonged compression with the tourniquet, lightheadedness after release of the tourniquet due to drug effects on blood pressure, and rarely, pulmonary embolism.

A variation of the nerve block technique also can be used to provide a more extended period of pain relief by destroying the nerves that contribute to the pain. When this is done, a needle is inserted close to the desired nerve or nerve bundle and an agent toxic to nerve, such as alcohol or phenol, is injected in place of the local anesthetic. After the procedure, neither motor nor sensory nerves are able to conduct impulses. The procedure leaves portions of the body incapable of sending a sensory signal to the spinal cord and free of any modifying influence that might be sent from the spinal cord. This technique has been used to treat conditions such as complex regional pain syndromes, in which the sympathetic nervous system sends nerve impulses to a region of the body and maintains a state of persistent pain. A reversible, diagnostic block of the sympathetic nervous system (*sympathetic block*) is performed as part of the initial evaluation. If pain relief is achieved, a permanent block may be attempted either through toxic injection or surgical intervention. These *neurolytic blocks*, while beneficial in some cases, fail to provide permanent relief in a large percentage of cases and, in some instances, lead to a worsening of the pain state. Recovery of functioning after a neurolytic injection can occur.

The next, more invasive procedures include the options for *nerve* and *spinal cord stimulation*. These procedures utilize varying levels of electrical stimulation delivered to those peripheral nerves or nerve bundles in the spinal cord that carry non-noxious signals. It is presumed that the increased level of activity in the stimulated nerves mimics the activity produced when one rubs or shakes an injured site on the body—it reduces the amount of pain signal transmitted to conscious levels of the brain. These stimulators are most effective for one-sided limb pain and are less effective for midline pain in the trunk and pelvis. Because psychological factors frequently contribute to stimulator failure, individuals must be appropriately screened for conditions that may decrease the likelihood of success. (Screening procedures are similar to those used prior to implantation of drug reservoirs and pumping systems for intrathecal delivery of medications, described in an earlier chapter.)

If psychological screening supports a stimulator trial, the individual is admitted to the hospital for implantation of the stimulating electrodes. Insulated wires carrying the electrical current, generated from a battery-powered stimulator, are inserted into the spinal canal through a catheter, in a fashion similar to inserting a needle to administer spinal anesthesia. The wires are positioned along the surface of the spinal cord in close proximity to the nerve bundles that convey non-noxious signals from the affected area, the dorsal columns. The wire's insulation is interrupted at intervals near its end to allow the current access to the nervous tissues. The other end of the wire is attached to a portable current source. For optimum electrode positioning, the individual receiving the implant must be awake during the procedure, to assist in guiding electrode placement and confirming a response to stimulation. On recovery, the individual is discharged from the hospital to complete the trial for several days in normal, familiar surroundings. The impact of stimulation on pain control is assessed for both beneficial and adverse effects. If successful, the individual then returns to the hospital for anchoring of the electrode wires and implantation beneath the skin of a permanent stimulator unit, a device about the size of a hockey puck. Stimulator output then may be controlled by a computerized instrument that can be placed over the power source. Although responsive individuals can experience significant reduction in their pain levels for several years, the need for medication may not always be eliminated. It should be noted that the analgesic effect from stimulation can diminish or be lost with time. This may be due to shifting of the electrodes from the site of placement or to the development of stimulation-induced scarring, similar to the formation of a protective callous on frequently irritated skin. The duration of effectiveness has increased significantly in recent years with the development of newer electrode systems. In addition, battery changes are required less frequently with the improvement of battery technology.

In the past, stimulator units also were attached to electrodes placed into structures deep in the brain, in an attempt to produce analgesia through stimulating the nerve cells that, when active, produce pain relief. These procedures required a neurosurgical opening of the skull and the anchoring of electrodes that were passed through brain in route to their target. Although pain relief was achieved in certain selected individuals, the results often were not permanent, likely because of electrode shifting and local scarring.

The most invasive procedures are those requiring general anesthesia and opening of the skin and body cavity. These procedures tend to be thought of early by the pain sufferer because of the perception that, in these days of advanced technologies and increased options, it should be possible to correct almost any ailment that arises. Although medical science has improved the quality of life for most people through advanced technology, there is still a long way to go before perception meets reality when it comes to pain control. From the perspective of the health care provider, surgical options are typically held until last, because of the irreversible nature of the process and the potential risks of infection, risks of failure, complications from anesthesia, and the possibility of unexpected injury. The potential for a good outcome not only depends on the skill of the surgeon, but on the condition of the person requiring the operation.

*Surgical procedures* are employed to remove any diseased or nonfunctional structures that compromise the function of adjacent tissues or to re-establish the integrity of a deformed or damaged structure. The desired result can be accomplished through surgical removal alone or with the introduction of natural tissue grafts or man-made devices in hopes of reducing pain and restoring function. In either case, the way the body redistributes forces imposed by gravity during activity are changed through alterations of the normal anatomy. Although such changes frequently lead to a finite period of improvement, they may be instrumental in the development of further problems at a later date. The duration of the beneficial effect is therefore important to consider when deciding whether to proceed with an operation. For an operation whose beneficial effect usually lasts for 5 years, if a good to excellent outcome is achieved in the majority of cases with minimal time in recovery and few complications, it may be prudent to consider this operation early in the case of someone suffering from cancer and whose life expectancy is less than 5 years. Conversely, if the operation loses its effect or worsens an underlying condition after the initial 5-year period of improvement, it may be unwise to consider the procedure for an otherwise healthy young adult who is likely to live for an additional 40 or 50 years. Each decision, however, must be made on a case-by-case basis to achieve the best result for each individual.

The problem of chronic *low back pain* provides an example to illustrate these issues when surgical intervention is an option. Low back pain is a complex problem that affects approximately 80% of the population at some time during their life. It is the second most common reason for an individual to seek counsel from a physician. Unfortunately, approximately 10% of those who suffer acute low back pain will develop a chronic condition. Despite the high incidence of back pain, the source of the noxious signal often is difficult to define. This may well be due to the variety of tissues in the back that are monitored by the nervous system to prevent injury, such as skin, muscles, tendons, ligaments, and bones, and the fact that most of these tissues are monitored by at least 3 levels of the spinal nerves. The overlap or redundancy in neuronal monitoring provides a back-up to insure protection and survival, but is an enigma for the physician attempting to procure an accurate diagnosis. Bulging or degenerative intervertebral disks can be found in many individuals who do not experience pain. Conversely, others experience pain at sites unrelated to the apparent pathology, and yet a third group of individuals experience pain in the absence of any obvious pathology. This variability provides a diagnostic dilemma when trying to decide whether and where to attempt to surgically correct a problem. In addition, episodes of back pain, even with anatomic evidence of a bulging disk, resolve without treatment in approximately 70% of individuals—and up to 24% of surgical procedures for back pain result in failure, with a 50% complication rate after disk removal. It is important, therefore, that surgical candidates are selected carefully and that the techniques to be considered (some of which are listed in Table 11-1) have been shown to be beneficial to reduce the incidence of postoperative problems and increase the likelihood of success. In general, operations performed solely to eliminate pain are likely to have a poor outcome, frequently result in an increased levels of pain, and have a poor prognosis for the future—including the need for additional operations to correct complications resulting from the first operation. By comparison, individuals suffering from pain associated with compromised nerve or spinal cord function are likely to realize a significant improvement in their pain and a preservation or return of neurologic function. Even with successful procedures, it is important to realize that total elimination of pain may not be achieved. The residual pain in successful cases typically responds better to conservative treatment options such as physical or occupational therapy and lower-strength analgesic medications.

When all other measures for pain control, tissue repair, or reconstruction have failed to produce adequate pain relief, *neurodestructive options* may be considered. In these procedures, portions of the pain pathways are destroyed by surgical transection, thermal coagulation, radiofrequency destruction (ablation), or radiation (gamma knife) to

**Table 11-1** Invasive Procedures for the Treatment of Back Pain

**Diskography**—A radiographic, diagnostic procedure to identify the source of persistent back pain in which an x-ray is obtained after an injection of a dye is made into the center of an intervertebral disc.

**Kyphoplasty**—A minimally invasive procedure designed to reduce pain and improve stability in which a balloon is inserted through a small incision into a compressed vertebra (fracture often seen in individuals with osteoporosis) and inflated to re-establish the height of the injured bone. The balloon is removed and replaced by a polymethylmethacrylate cement to provide stability.

**Vertebroplasty**—Similar to kyphoplasty, but without the insertion of the balloon.

Intradiscal Electorthermal Therapy (IDET)—A minimally invasive procedure in which a heating wire is inserted through a guide needle that has been inserted into an injured vertebral disc. The wire is then heated to slowly cauterize nerve endings in the outer portion of the disc and to solidify the gelatinous center of the disc, like hard boiling an egg, and then removed.

**Diskectomy**—The surgical removal of all (total) or part (partial) of a bulging (herniated) disc in order to preserve function and reveal pain associated with pressure placed on nerve roots or spinal cord.

**Vertebral Fusion**—The surgical stabilization of portions of the spinal column after disc removal through grafting bone harvested from cadavers or from another portion of the individual undergoing fusion (often from the crest of the hip bone) in order to re-establish structural stability.

**Disc Replacement**—The replacement of damaged intervertebral disc with prosthetic devises designed to re-establish anatomical stability while retaining some flexibility similar to normal function.

**Pedicular Screws, Stabilization Rods, and Plates**—Surgical implantable supportive elements used to re-establish vertebral stability when biological elements are insufficient, due to structural inadequacies or the extent of the damage needing repair.

block the noxious signal from reaching conscious levels. To relieve pain from a limited region of the body, specific peripheral nerves may be cut (*neurectomy* or *neurotomy*) to remove a site of spontaneous activity. Sensory nerves generally are considered reasonable candidates for neurectomy because their destruction does not significantly impair motor function. If larger areas of analgesia are necessary, the dorsal roots of one or several selected spinal nerves may be cut (*dorsal rhizotomy or dorsal root entry zone [DREZ] destruction*) close to their entry into the spinal cord. Although the neuronal pathways involved provide a purely sensory function, the damage is not restricted to pain fibers alone. Loss of neurons that monitor muscle length and joint position are compromised as well, which leads to impairment of motor coordination. This type of procedure has been shown to be effective in treating some cases of trigeminal neuralgia and, with careful destruction of only selected nerve roots, prolonged benefit may be achieved. If very large portions of the body, such as the entire left trunk below the navel and the left leg, are involved with pain, transection of the lateral spinothalamic tract in the spinal cord (*myelotomy*) at the appropriate level will produce analgesia to the entire region. Because information about non-noxious stimulation is transmitted through fiber bundles that course through a different portion of the spinal cord than do the pain fibers, these procedures preserve normal non-noxious sensation. Finally, procedures have been performed (although very infrequently) to destroy portions of the cerebral hemispheres thought to be involve in pain processing (*cingulotomy*). These procedures seem to reduce the emotional and subjective quality of pain without eliminating its perception—the needle stick is there, but the "Ouch" is gone. Although these procedures produce profound analgesia in most cases, the effect is often transient. Pain frequently returns, often at increased levels, months to years after surgery. Individuals with predictable short-term survival may be excellent candidates for such procedures. Probable long-term survivors who suffer from neuropathic pain conditions, however, may be well-advised to proceed with caution. These patients have already demonstrated a propensity for developing neuropathic pain, and it is not unlikely that additional injury to neural structures at the surgical sites may ultimately lead to increased pain.

CHAPTER 12

# Age and Sex—Special Considerations for Pain Management

T HE GENERAL PRINCIPLES of pain perception and the principles that guide pain management apply to all who suffer and to all who play a role in treating pain. However, recent investigations have begun to appreciate that certain conditions may require special consideration if maximum benefit from treatment is to be achieved. Perhaps the most important of these conditions relates to age and sex.

## CONSIDERATIONS FOR PAIN IN CHILDREN

Only in the last 15 years has there been an appreciation that the pain pathways are sufficiently developed at the time of birth to receive noxious stimuli and to convey signals perceived as painful by the newborn child. Prior to this revelation, painful procedures such as circumcisions, repeated heel sticks to obtain blood samples and, at a somewhat later age, hypodermic injections and venipuncture, were routinely performed on newborns and young children without the benefit of anesthetic. The perception was that, since the pain pathways were not completely developed at birth, pain was not perceived and therefore such procedures would have no effect on the child in later years. In the context of what is currently known about the developing nervous system, however, it is not unlikely that uncontrolled pain perceived soon after birth and in early childhood may have a very profound effect on the way pain is perceived and appreciated at later ages. In the early stages of postnatal development, the nervous system begins to interact with the complex world around it. It is in a position to receive stimuli from the environment and, during certain critical periods of time after birth, can respond to these stimuli in such a way that neuronal circuits are modified to improve processing at a later date. In other words, an event is entered on an empty slate for later reference. As the individual ages, the ability to make such changes decreases; some opportunities never recur, but changes made are never lost. Changes in the nervous system that occur in response to an early unpleasant painful event may even influence how one approaches prophylactic health care as an adult. This may be the case with individuals who experienced dental procedures without benefit of lidocaine, and who continue to cringe at the sound of a dental drill and are reluctant to avail themselves of routine dental check-ups for reasons that are "unclear." It is therefore important to realize that most pain perceived early in development is perceived similarly to the way it is perceived by adults. Pain therefore should be recognized when it is present at all ages, and it should be managed appropriately, particularly in children, to prevent later problems.

Because children are unable to report pain due to lack of verbal skills, it falls to the care giver to be observant and recognized nonverbal behavior that is consistent with the perception of pain. In newborns, high-pitched cries associated with facial grimacing, body rigidity, and withdrawal are indicators of pain. These behaviors can be contrasted with the crying associated with facial expressions of sadness during anxiety and with the clutching of toys, blankets, and parents during separation. For older children, pain intensity can be assessed through the use of color or picture scales that are selected in accordance with the child's communicative abilities. Despite the lack of verbal skills, with observation, it may actually be easier to accurately assess pain in young children due to the lack of confounding issues associated with secondary gain. Secondary gain may include avoiding an unpleasant activity or winning the additional attention of a parent. Secondary issues related to school activities such as postponing an exam to get more time to study, however, should be considered as a possible contributing factor in the presentation of a pain complaint in school-aged children.

Issues not frequently considered during the evaluation of an adult may have a profound influence on a similar experience for a child. If recognized and addressed, corrective measures suitable for age may reduce the painful experience. Comfortable surroundings, enriched with non-noxious stimuli, tend to reduce anxiety and distract the child from objects that might otherwise appear threatening. Depending on age and situation, the presence of parents or siblings may modify the response to a potentially painful experience either positively by reducing anxiety or negatively by providing a source for possible secondary gain. A pleasant attitude and the friendly appearance of the health care providers also can provide a sense of trust and reassurance through nonverbal cues.

Although nonpharmacologic treatment options should be employed when appropriate, and the use of noninvasive treatments are preferred, the use of medications is still an important part of the pain-relieving armamentarium for children. It is important to realize, however, that children are not just small adults. The metabolism of some medications differs in children, and adjustments must be made to achieve maximum success at different developmental stages. Several therapeutic options have a special role for the management of pain in children. One such option for the very young, between birth and about 5 months of age, is that sucrose, in conjunction with suckling, has been shown to be beneficial in relieving pain. After 5 months, this benefit is lost, and other options must be considered. Second, the use of acetaminophen for treatment of pain related to mild to moderate musculoskeletal pain and fever is especially relevant in children, because the use of aspirin for fever, especially associated with viral infections, puts the child at risk for developing Reye syndrome, a condition associated with mental confusion, brain swelling, low blood sugar, impaired liver function, and seizures. Complications from Reye syndrome can be devastating, leading to central nervous system damage and death. However, when pain is related to inflammation associated with trauma, nonsteroidal anti-inflammatory agents (NSAIDs) are preferred. In the event that invasive procedures, such as hypodermic injection, venipuncture, and skin biopsy, are necessary, pretreatment of the area with topical prilocaine and lidocaine (EMLA) significantly decreases the discomfort associated with injections and the use of surgical instruments.

## CONSIDERATIONS FOR PAIN IN THE ELDERLY

Special considerations also must be made when treating pain at the other end of the age spectrum. Many of the differences encountered are related to the aging process in general and considerations of end-of-life issues, yet others seem to be related more to lack of knowledge about pain's role in the natural process of aging. Unfortunately, many of these issues have resulted in inadequate reporting of pain, subsequent insufficient pain assessment and management, and a significant reduction in quality of life during the later years.

The misconceptions about pain in the elderly are numerous and varied, but not always obvious, because the individual who is suffering the increased frequency of pain may view it as natural and appropriate to the aging process, and his health care provider dutifully accepts conditions at their face value in the context of busy schedules. One misconception, therefore, is that pain is just a part of old age. Many believe that pain is to be expected, is perceived as not valid to report and, in most cases, must be endured. In conjunction with this perception, most individuals do not wish to be viewed as constant complainers. To be viewed as a "good patient," complaints about "expected" pain often are kept to a minimum. Health care providers reinforce this conception through the belief that pain is perceived less intensely in the elderly, and these providers do not ask about or look for signs of discomfort. Fortunately, in recent years, with the increased focus on exercise, rest, and good nutrition, pain occurring in the elderly has shifted more to the eighth and ninth decade of life, but is more closely correlated to *physical age* (determined by overall health status), rather than chronologic age (determined by birth date). This observation supports the preemptive management of potential pain problems by nonpharmacologic means through physical conditioning.

Another misconception is that pain is a consequence of living a less than perfect life. Pain thus is not reported because the individual perceives it as something deserved—pain must be endured as penance for earlier transgressions.

Other individuals choose not to report their pain because they fear that the initiation of pain treatment, especially in later life, marks the beginning of their death. This perception often is correlated with prior experiences, in which the initiation of pain treatment closely preceded the death of a relative or friend.

Another misconception that leads to less reporting of pain in the elderly is related to the individual's increased awareness of their mortality and an underlying concern about the mechanism of their death. In this context, pain may be perceived as the harbinger of death, and it goes unreported because its existence is denied. Others do not report their pain because they fear increased pain related to possible diagnostic testing that may be incurred and the treatments that may be imposed. Still others may be concerned about the medication side effects that they may have to endure and the potential for addiction.

Because of senility, adverse effects of medications, and disease, the elderly may have difficulty communicating their discomfort and need for pain control. In these situations, alternative methods for pain assessment must be considered. In some instances, assessment is possible using the same pain-measuring tools used for children. The practitioner must be prepared, however, to observe behavior and interpret mood changes and facial expression as possible indicators of pain intensity. These issues are important to consider because untreated, unrelenting pain frequently leads to depression, sleep problems, a reduction in the ability to walk and perform personal activities of daily living, and decreased socialization with friends and family—a vicious, downhill, reinforcing spiral that decreases the quality of life.

General consequences of the aging process also play a role in the amount of pain experienced by elderly individuals. In general, the elderly are more susceptible to injury as a result of the presence of stiffer, less compliant muscles, tendons, and ligaments; decreases in bone density that increase the risk of fracture; and decreased response to unexpected threats, such as uneven floors and sidewalks. When injury occurs, recuperation is slower due to a decline in regenerative capacity. Elderly individuals also experience more medical problems that are likely to produce pain, related in part to a decline in the immune system's ability to fight disease. In addition, the elderly are likely to be taking a wider variety of medications than are younger adults. This constellation of circumstances increases the likelihood that, in the later stages of life, pain is likely to be present at some level for a greater portion of the elderly age group, the spectrum of causes for pain is broader than in younger adults, and a greater potential exists for treatment complications as a result of medication interactions. Some concurrent treatments may reduce the effect of some analgesic regimens through shifts in drug absorption and breakdown. Conversely, some pain treatments may increase or decrease the effects of treatments for other pre-existing problems. Thus, when seeking treatment for pain, it is especially important for elderly individuals to report all concurrent medical conditions and medications, including home remedies and over-the-counter preparations, to increase the likelihood of satisfactory treatment and reduce the risk of drug complications. Home remedies and over-the-counter preparations frequently are used to reduce pain and thereby decrease the need "to complain" to the health care provider. The use of such remedies seldom is reported, although they may have a significant effect on treatment outcome and must be considered.

As with other patients, a good rule for treatment of pain in the elderly is to "start low and go slow." Some treatments that produce little or no adverse effects in a young adult may have profound effects in someone who has a lower body mass and whose physiologic status influences absorption, distribution, and breakdown of drugs and alters the expected properties of a medication.

As in the treatment of all individuals, intermittent, acute pain should be treated as needed. If possible, treat in anticipation of pain usually associated with scheduled stressful events, like travel and certain planned activities. Acetaminophen is the drug of choice in the elderly for mild to moderate musculoskeletal pain, because NSAIDs may significantly alter blood pressure, produce gastrointestinal problems and fluid retention, and compromise kidney function. When necessary, the course of treatment with NSAIDs should be short-term and should include liver and kidney function monitoring. The risk of complication increases significantly when high doses and multiple nonsteroidal preparations are used in combination.

For chronic pain, sustained-release preparations should be provided on the clock to maximize coverage and reduce the need for higher doses of medication. Prophylactic treatment for constipation should be initiated with all treatment regimens that utilize opioid preparations. This is especially true in the elderly, since dietary changes, both in the types of foods that are tolerated and the regularity of the times and amounts of food that are consumed, often lead to constipation even in those who are not taking opioid medications. In all instances, adjuvant medications should be considered, but caution must be exercised when using multiple central nervous system depressants, because the sedating effects may be excessive, thereby limiting activity and increasing the risk of injury due to falls.

## End-of-Life Issues

Not just for the elderly, but for all those dealing with terminal disease, it is important to remember that psychosocial issues contribute significantly to the perception of pain. Concerns about end-of-life issues play a major role in pain management and quality of life. From a practical perspective, the consideration of a patient's wishes for interventions, such as the use of ventilators and cardiac resuscitation in the case of heart or lung failure, should be addressed early. Completion of wills and plans for disposition of worldly remains well ahead of death also frees the individual from concern about unfinished business. From the perspective of the health care provider, it is important to recognize potential psychological issues and provide assistance when necessary in the form of counseling and social services. Attention to the psychosocial details reduces anxiety both for the patient and the family, reduces the psychological stresses that can enhance pain perception, and allows for more quality time when it is most important.

## GENDER CONSIDERATIONS FOR PAIN ASSESSMENT AND TREATMENT

Although some significant strides have been made toward improving equality for women in education, sports, and the workplace, recognizing *"la difference"* may be a better approach when it comes to pain management. Recent efforts to recognize the special needs and concerns of women in relation to health care have identified several important gender distinctions related to the perception and treatment of pain. These distinctions can be attributed to many factors, including sex-linked genetic differences that convey a different susceptibility to various diseases and response to medication; anatomic differences that can define risks for potential injury; hormonal differences that play a role in drug metabolism, the vigilance of the immune system, and response to trauma; and differences in the ability to cope with stress.

Research shows that women report pain at stimulus intensities typically lower than those that produce pain in men. In addition, women tolerate pain less well, are more likely to report pain at higher intensity levels, and are more likely to report pain than men. An exception, and indeed a reversal, to this general observation is seen when noxious stimulation is administered to men in the region of the lower abdomen and genitalia. Coupled with the greater propensity to perceive and report pain, women are presented with a wider variety of naturally occurring painful conditions, such as monthly menstrual pain, pregnancy, childbirth, and menopause, and are more susceptible to a greater number of painful diseases. Migraine headaches, fibromyalgia, irritable bowel syndrome, rheumatoid arthritis, and multiple sclerosis occur much more frequently in women than in men. Fortunately, the overwhelming predisposition for women to experience pain is counterbalanced by a greater willingness to seek assistance and to try different treatment options. Women also have a greater ability to cope with the pain, perhaps due to the frequency with which it is perceived.

Anatomic differences also contribute to the frequency of perceiving pain. The internal location of sexual organs, which are highly innervated by the pain-predominating C-fiber system, increases the volume of pelvic contents for women compared to men. Diseases and trauma involving the internal sexual organs thus are in a position to influence adjacent internal structures, making differential diagnosis of low back, abdominal, and pelvic pain more extensive than in men, whose sexual organs are externally placed. Even secondary sexual features related to breast development can affect posture and ultimately contribute to problems of low back pain.

In addition, genetically determined gender differences evident in the constellation of neural receptors in the brain can ultimately influence the response to certain opioid and anxiety-reducing medications; this factor may provide additional treatment options for women. This is illustrated by the observation that nalbuphine, buprenorphine, and pentazocine, all of which have special affinity for a specific subtype of opioid receptor prevalent in women, produce greater pain relief than morphine in women than they do in men.

Basal body functions, including growth and healing, metabolism of nutrients and the utilization of energy, adjustment of fluid levels, and reproductive survival are governed by hormones that circulate through the body and affect the function of every organ system. From a health care perspective, hormones also influence the ability of the immune system to fight disease and regulate the absorption and metabolism of drugs. Women experience greater fluctuations in hormones throughout their life than do men. These fluctuations are related to puberty; the menstrual cycle throughout reproductive life with additional alterations in hormonal excursions related to pregnancy, birth, and postpartum changes; menopause; and senescence. Because hormonal balance shifts throughout the menstrual cycle, fluid balance, drug absorption, distribution, metabolism, clearance, and excretion (as well as a woman's response to painful stimuli) increase or decrease, regularly or irregularly, from a predicted level that depends on the phase of the cycle for that month. Hormonal changes, therefore, are likely to influence the effectiveness and perhaps the safety of medications taken at different times during the menstrual cycle. This variation is likely to explain the fluctuations in pain complaints, reports of capricious variation in pain control, and adverse effects reported by women while on a routine treatment regimen.

Although gender differences always have been present, the greater realization of the magnitude of these differences and how they affect pain perception and treatment may well lead to improved care. As more is understood about the gender differences in pain, the most effective treatment plans will begin to include adjustments of medications, or perhaps adjustments of hormones, based on the phase of life and the phase of the menstrual cycle. This may enable health care providers to prescribe a selection of medications that take advantage of gender-specific receptors in the brain and to increase the implementation of alternative treatments and interventions to improve pain control.

The recognition of age and gender differences in the pain experience re-emphasizes the theme that I have tried to convey throughout this book: Pain is different for every person experiencing it. It thus must be evaluated completely in each case and for each individual, and a treatment regimen that addresses the multifactorial nature of pain must be tailored to fit each particular patient, if success in pain control and improvement in quality of life is to be attained. Unfortunately, even in the best of all situations, in this day and age, times remain when all efforts to relieve pain are unsuccessful. It is my hope that, through continued research, inquiry, education, and investigation, the number of patients failing to find relief will progressively decrease and that none of these cases will be due to a lack of understanding, caring, or compassion.

# Glossary

**A-beta (αβ) system**
Large diameter, rapidly conducting axons that convey signals related to light touch.

**A-delta (αδ) system**
The smallest myelinated axons that rapidly convey signals related to noxious stimulation.

**Action potential**
Electrical impulse or nerve signal conducted by an axon.

**Acute pain**
Pain that occurs at the time of an injury and lasts for only that period of time when the reason for the pain is present.

**Addiction**
The psychological dependence on any substance taken for the psychological benefits that are derived, irrespective of therapeutic necessity and despite effects that are identified and found to be deleterious.

**Adjuvant medications**
Drugs with analgesic properties that were designed to treat a condition other than pain.

**Afferents**
Elements conducting information into the central nervous system.

**Agonist**
A drug that combines with a receptor to initiate an effect.

**Allodynia**
The perception of pain resulting from non-painful stimulation.

**Analgesic**
Pain-relieving.

**Analgesic ceiling**
Dosage of a particular drug above which no additional pain relief can be achieved.

**Antagonist**
A drug that opposes the effect of an agonist.

**Anticonvulsant agents**
Drugs used to treat epilepsy (recurrent seizures).

**Antidepressant agents**
Drugs used to treat depression.

**Antihypertensive agents**
Drugs used to treat blood pressure.

**Antispasmodic agents**
Drugs used to treat muscle spasm.

**Autonomic nervous system**
The part of the peripheral nervous system that deals with functions not consciously controlled, e.g., heart rate, size of blood vessels, breathing rate, and intestinal movements.

**Axon**
The conducting portion of the nerve cell.

**C-fiber system**
Smallest diameter, unmyelinated axons that slow conduct axon signals related to noxious stimulation.

**Category scale**
A method used to record pain intensity in which a series of words, e.g., mild, discomforting, distressing, horrible, and excruciating are used to describe different pain levels.

**Central nervous system (CNS)**
Brain and spinal cord.

**Central pain**
Pain that occurs as a result of central nervous system injury.

**Cerebral cortex**
The "thinking" portion of the brain that analyzes sensory information in association with past experience and formulates a behavioral response.

**Cervical vertebra**
One of seven bones of the spinal column found in the neck.

**Chemotherapy**
Chemical or drug treatment for a disease.

**Chronic pain**
Pain that occurs for prolonged periods of time.

**Cognitive therapy**
Brain initiated control.

**Coronary artery**
Arterial vessel that carries blood to the heart muscle.

**Dependency**
An adaptive phenomenon in which cells of the body alter their normal function to accommodate for repetitive exposure to certain regularly taken substances.

**Depolarization**
Equilibration of charge across an axonal membrane that results in the generation of an action potential.

**Dorsal column**
A bundle of axons within the spinal cord that conducts information about light touch, vibration, and position sense.

**Dorsal column stimulation**
A method for producing pain control in which electrical current is administered through implanted electrodes to the dorsal columns of the spinal cord.

**Dorsal horn**
A collection of nerve cell bodies inside the spinal cord that receive signals from peripheral sensory neurons (peripheral afferents).

**Dorsal rhizotomy (dorsal root entry zone [DREZ] destruction)**
Cutting the dorsal root prior to its entry into the spinal cord.

**Dorsal root**
Sensory nerve axons that enter the spinal cord.

**Dorsal root ganglion**
A collection of sensory neuronal cell bodies located along the course of the dorsal root.

**Ectopic**
Abnormally positioned.

**Efferents**
Elements conducting information away from the central nervous system.

**Endorphins**
Opioid-like chemicals produced by the brain.

**Faces pain or "Oucher" scale**
A method used to record pain intensity in which a series of cartoon faces that depict a smiling face at the "No Pain" end and a face that is crying at the "Worst Pain" end.

**Facticious pain**
Pain that is fabricated for personal gain, reward, or satisfaction.

**Focal pain**
Pain that is located in a restricted region of the body.

**Free nerve endings**
Nerve endings associated with neurons that receive noxious chemical, thermal, and mechanical stimulation.

**Ganglion**
A collection of nerve cell bodies located outside the central nervous system.

**Golgi tendon organ**
A specialized sensory nerve ending designed to detect and protect a muscle from excessive stretch.

**Hernia**
Protrusion of contained tissues through the wall of the confining structure; as in the spine, the protrusion of soft disk material through the wall of the intervertebral disk ("slipped disk").

**Hypothalamus**
The portion of the brain stem that monitors basic body functions such as thirst, hunger, satiety, sexual function, blood pressure, temperature, and emotion.

**Idiopathic pain**
Pain complaints that defy the diagnostic skills of the healthcare provider and are not characterized as nociceptive, neuropathic, or psychogenic in origin.

**Inflammation**
The process associated with clean-up and repair of injured tissue.

**Interferential stimulation**
Electrical stimulation that produces analgesia by stimulating large, low threshold nerve cells with deeper penetration of the tissue than available with TENS.

**Intervertebral disk**
Tissue between the vertebrae of the spinal column that provides cushioning and allows limited movement between vertebrae.

**Intrathecal infusion**
Drug administered directly into the spinal fluid via a subcutaneously implanted pump and catheter system.

**Ion channels**
Protein pores in the nerve cell membrane that open and close in response to stimulus to allow passage of charged particles (ions), e.g., sodium, calcium, potassium, in and out of the nerve cell.

**Iontophoretic delivery system**
Medication is delivered through the skin using low-level electrical current.

**Lateral spinothalamic tract**
A bundle of axons within the spinal cord that conducts information about noxious stimulation.

**Lumbar vertebra**
One of five bones of the spinal column found in the low back.

**Malingering**
Pain that is fabricated for personal gain, reward, or satisfaction.

**Mechanisms**
Processes underlying function.

**Medial lemniscus**
A bundle of axons within the brain stem that conducts information about light touch, vibration, and position sense.

**Medulla**
A region of the brain stem.

**Meissner's corpuscle**
A specialized sensory nerve ending designed to detect pressure.

**Merkel cell**
A specialized sensory nerve ending designed to detect light touch.

**Modulation**
Positive or negative adjustment of neuronal activity.

**Multidisciplinary**
More that one specialty.

**Multifaceted**
Complex, involving many components.

**Multifocal pain**
Pain that is felt in more than one part of the body.

**Myelin**
The insulating covering of an axon.

**Myelotomy**
Transection of the lateral spinothalamic tract to produce regional analgesia.

**Nerve block**
Injection or infiltration of a local anesthetic in close proximity to a nerve that blocks conduction of the nerve.

**Neurodestructive procedure**
A procedure that produces analgesia through the destruction of a nerve or neural pathway.

**Neurectomy (neurotomy)**
Cutting of a peripheral nerve.

**Neurolytic block**
Permanent nerve block achieved by injection or infiltration of a toxin in close proximity to a nerve.

**Neuropathic pain**
Pain that is associated with injury to either the brain and spinal cord or the peripheral nerves that results in abnormal activity of the nervous system and may be present in the absence of any ongoing tissue injury.

**Neurotransmitters**
Chemicals released by nerve cell terminals that are responsible for relaying information from one nerve cell to another.

**Nociceptive pain**
Pain that is associated with actual or potential tissue injury in the presence of a normally functioning nervous system.

**Node of Ranvier**
Gap in the myelin sheath of an axon that is associated with the most excitable portion of the axon.

**Noxious stimulus**
A stimulus sufficient to cause an uncomfortable sensation and potentially damage tissue.

**Nucleus gigantocellularis**
A collection of neurons in the brain stem associated with the descending pathways that modify the pain signal in the dorsal horn as it enters the spinal cord.

**Nucleus raphe magnus**
A collection of neurons in the brain stem associated with the descending pathways that modify the pain signal in the dorsal horn as it enters the spinal cord.

**Numeric rating scale (NRS)**
A method used to record pain intensity in which intensity is indicated by numbers that range between 0 and 10 where 0 represents no pain and 10 represents the worst pain imagined based on past experience.

**Opioid medications**
Alkaloid analgesic medications that are either derived naturally from opium, modified or synthesized in the laboratory.

**Pacinian corpuscle**
A specialized sensory nerve ending designed to detect vibration.

**Pain**
A sensory and emotional experience that is associated with actual or potential tissue injury and is described in such terms.

**Parasympathetic nervous system**
The part of the autonomic nervous system that is active during vegetative or rejuvenative periods of life and serves to enhance digestion and restfulness.

**Patient-controlled analgesia (PCA)**
Drug administration technology that provides constant infusion of analgesic medication and the possibility for delivery of predetermined, on-demand dosing for breakthrough pain.

**Periaqueductal grey**
A collection of neurons in the brain stem associated with the descending pathways that modify the pain signal in the dorsal horn as it enters the spinal cord.

**Peripheral nervous system (PNS)**
Nervous system structures, nerves, which convey signals to and from the central nervous system to the body wall and its contents.

**Pseudoaddiction**
Seeking of additional medications for inadequately treated pain.

**Psychogenic pain**
Pain that results from emotional conflict or psychological problems that are sufficient to allow the conclusion that they are the main causative influence.

**Radiating pain**
Pain that spreads from an initial focus to another portion of the body.

**Recurrent acute pain**
Pain that occur regularly.

**Referred pain**
Pain resulting from a focal injury felt in a location distant from the site of tissue injury.

**Regional anesthesia**
Isolated intravenous administration of drug to produce anesthesia for an entire limb.

**Sacrum**
A single bone, derived from the natural fusion of five vertebra during development, in the pelvic region of the spinal column.

**Schwann cell**
Cell that supports axons and produces myelin, the insulating covering of the axon.

**Sensory neurons**
Nerve cells that receive sensory information and transmit a signal to the central nervous system.

**Somatic pain**
Pain that is associated with structures of the body wall, e.g., skin, muscles, and bones.

**Spindle organ**
A specialized sensory nerve ending designed to detect fine differences in muscle stretch.

**Subtherapeutic range**
Medication levels insufficient to produce the desired effect.

**Sympathetic nervous system**
The part of the autonomic nervous system that prepares the body for "fight or flight."

**Synapse**
A specialized structure between nerve cells where normal impulses are passed from one cell to another.

**Synaptic cleft**
The space between two nerve cells within a synapse which neurotransmitters must cross to convey an impulse.

**Transcutaneous electrical nerve stimulation (TENS)**
Electrical stimulation that produces analgesia by stimulating large, relatively superficial, low threshold nerve cells.

**Transdermal delivery system**
Medication is delivered in a controlled fashion through the skin from an externally applied reservoir and filtering patch.

**Thalamus**
A collection of neuronal cell bodies within the brain stem that serves as the final relay station for information coming from the body en route to the cerebral cortex.

**Therapeutic range**
Medication levels that produce the desired effect.

**Thoracic vertebra**
One of 12 bones of the spinal column found in the chest each associated with a rib.

**Tolerance**
Loss of medication effect over time.

**Topical agents**
Medications applied to the skin.

**Toxic range**
Medication levels that produce the adverse effects.

**Ventral root**
Motor nerve axons that leave the spinal cord.

**Visceral pain**
Pain that is associated with visceral organs, e.g., stomach, intestine, liver, and pancreas.

**Visual analogue scale (VAS)**
A method used to record pain intensity in which the intensity is indicated by a mark along a line that represents the range of intensity from "No Pain" at one end of the line to "Worst Pain" at the other.

**Wind-up**

A phenomenon associated with repetitive C-fiber activity in which there is a perception of stimulus increase irrespective of an increase in stimulus intensity.

**Withdrawal**

Symptoms associated with the rapid discontinuation of a dependency-producing medication.

# Resources

## General Pain Issues

**American Pain Society**
4700 W. Lake Avenue
Glenview, IL 60025
Phone: 847-375-4715
Fax: 877-734-8758 [Toll Free]
E-mail: info@ampainsoc.org
Website: http://www.ampainsoc.org

The American Pain Society is a multidisciplinary organization of basic and clinical scientists, practicing clinicians, policy analysts, and others. The mission of the American Pain Society is to advance pain-related research, education, treatment, and professional practice. This site offers features for health care professionals and educational materials for the general public.

**American Academy of Pain Medicine**
4700 W. Lake Avenue
Glenview, IL 60025
Phone: 847-375-4731
Fax: 877-734-8750
E-mail: aapm@amctec.com
Website: http://www.painmed.org

The American Academy of Pain Medicine (AAPM) is the medical-specialty society representing physicians practicing in the field of pain medicine. As a medical-specialty society, the academy is involved in education, training, advocacy, and research in the specialty of pain medicine.

## American Board of Pain Medicine

4700 W. Lake Avenue

Glenview, IL 60025

Phone: 847-375-4726

Fax: 877-734-8751

Website: http://www.abpm.org

The mission of the American Board of Pain Medicine is to serve the public by improving the quality of pain medicine, to evaluate candidates who voluntarily appear for examination, and to certify as Diplomates in Pain Medicine those who are qualified; to maintain and improve the quality of graduate medical education in the field of pain medicine by collaborating with related organizations; and to provide information about the specialty of pain medicine to the public.

## The National Initiative on Pain Control

Website: http://www.painedu.org

The National Initiative on Pain Control (NIPC) is dedicated to helping physicians and other health care professionals better understand the need for appropriate pain management.

## American Society of Addiction Medicine

Website: http://www.asam.org/pain/pain_and_addiction_medicine

The mission of the Pain Committee of the Society for Pain and Addiction Medicine is to encourage collaboration, including research, education, clinical practice, and policy initiatives, between pain specialists and addiction specialists on issues of common interest related to pain and addiction.

## University of Wisconsin Pain and Policy Studies Group (PPSG)

Pain & Policy Studies Group

406 Science Drive, Suite 202

Madison, WI 53711-1068

Phone: 608-263-7662

E-mail: ppsg@med.wisc.edu

Website: http://www.medsch.wisc.edu/painpolicy

The purpose of this website is to facilitate public access to information about pain relief and public policy, including material published by the PPSG and other authoritative sources. The intended audiences for this information include patients, the public, and professionals in medicine, pharmacy, nursing, palliative care, cancer care, law, and other related disciplines. The Pain & Policy Studies Group, at the University of Wisconsin, addresses both domestic and international policy issues and is a World Health Organization Collaborating Center for Policy and Communications in Cancer Care.

**International Association for the Study of Pain**
IASP Secretariat
909 NE 43rd Street, Suite 306
Seattle, WA 98105-6020
Phone: 206-547-6409
Fax: 206-547-1703
E-mail: iaspdesk@iasp-pain.org
Website: http://www.isap-pain.org and http://www.painbooks.org

The International Association is multidisciplinary and is open to all professionals involved in the research and treatment of all types of pain including acute pain, chronic pain, and cancer pain and others.

**American Pain Foundation**
201 North Charles Street, Suite 710
Baltimore, Maryland 21201-4111
Phone: 888-615-7246
Website: http://www.painfoundation.org

Provides resources for patients, families, health care professionals, and legislators related to pain issues.

**American Chronic Pain Association**
The ACPA
P.O. Box 850
Rocklin, CA 95677
Phone: 1-800-533-3231

Fax: 916-632-3208

Website: http://www.theapca.org

The mission of the American Board of Pain Medicine is to facilitate peer support and education for individuals with chronic pain and their families so that these individuals may live more fully in spite of their pain; and to raise awareness among the health care community, policy makers, and the public at large about issues of living with chronic pain. The ACPA offers support and information for people with chronic pain.

## Partners Against Pain

One Stamford Forum

Stamford, CT 06901-3431

Phone: 888-726-7535; at message, please press "5" for Partners Against Pain inquiries.

E-mail: partnersagainstpain@pharma.com

Website: http://www.partnersagainstpain.com

Partners Against Pain is an alliance of patients, caregivers, and health care providers working together to alleviate unnecessary suffering by leading efforts to advance standards of pain care through education and advocacy.

## CANCER PAIN

Cancer-Pain.org

Website: http://www.cancer-pain.org

Cancer-pain.org has been developed by the Association of Cancer Online Resources with input and advice from patients, caregivers, and an Advisory Board of health care professionals dedicated to providing the most advanced cancer pain relief. Their aim is to help cancer patients receive the pain treatment they deserve.

## American Cancer Society

Phone: 1-800-ACS-2345

Website: http://www.cancer.org

The American Cancer Society is the nationwide community-based voluntary health organization dedicated to eliminating cancer as a major health problem by preventing cancer, saving lives, and diminishing suffering from cancer, through research, education, advocacy, and service.

## NEUROLOGICAL ISSUES

### American Academy of Neurology
1080 Montreal Avenue
Saint Paul, MN 55116
Website: http://www.aan.com

The American Academy of Neurology is an organization of neurology professionals whose website serves its membership with educational materials to aid in patient care. Patient education can be obtained by accessing the affiliate site www.thebrainmatters.org .

### The Neuropathy Association
The Neuropathy Association, Inc.
P.O. Box 26226
New York, NY 10117-3422
Phone: 212-692-0662
E-mail: info@neuropathy.org
Website: http://www.neuropathy.org

The Neuropathy Association provides information and support to help better understand this neurologic disorder and how to cope with it. The association is committed to raising the awareness of peripheral neuropathy and supporting the research to find its cure.

### American Council for Headache Education
19 Nautua Road
Mt. Royal, NJ 08061
Phone: 856-423-0258; 1-800-255-2243
Fax: 856-423-0082
E-mail: achehq@talley.com
Website: http://www.ahsnet.org

This organization, in conjunction with the *American Headache Society*, is dedicated to the treatment and management of headache, and provides educational information for the individuals and families of those suffering with headache.

## WOMEN'S PAIN ISSUES

### International Pelvic Pain Society
1080 Montreal Avenue
Saint Paul, MN 55116
Phone: 205-877-2950 or 1-800-624-9676 if in the U.S.
Website: http://www.pelvicpain.org

The goals of the International Pelvic Pain Society are to serve as an educational resource for health care professionals, to optimize diagnosis and treatment of patients suffering from chronic pelvic pain, to collate research in chronic pelvic pain, to inform women, and to serve as a resource of education for treatment options and professional health care members.

### National Fibromyalgia Association (NFA)
2200 N. Glassell Street, Suite A
Orange, CA 92865
Phone: 714-921-0150
Fax: 714-921-6920
Website: http://www.fmaware.org

The National Fibromyalgia Association (previously known as the National Fibromyalgia Awareness Campaign) is a nonprofit organization whose mission is to develop and execute programs dedicated to improving the quality of life for people with fibromyalgia by increasing the awareness of the public, media, government, and medical communities. The NFA provides patient information and education through international conferences, regional seminars, brochures, informational handouts, video and audio tapes, newsletters, a website, telephone assistance, and online advice, giving patients one-on-one help. It also publishes the *Fibromyalgia Aware* magazine three times a year and provides continuing education programs for health care professionals.

**National Vulvodynia Association**
P.O. Box 4491
Silver Spring, MD 20914-4491
Phone: 301-299-0775
Fax: 301-299-3999
Website: http://www.nva.org

The National Vulvodynia Association is a nonprofit organization created to improve the lives of individuals affected by vulvodynia, a spectrum of chronic vulvar pain disorders. The association provides education for affected women about the disease, current treatments and resources for treatment, encouragement to develop self-help strategies to deal with the physical and emotional components of this disorder, and a network of support for family and those suffering with the disease.

## CHILDREN'S PAIN ISSUES

**American Academy of Pediatrics**
141 Northwest Point Boulevard
Elk Grove Village, IL, 60007
Phone: 847-434-4000
Fax: 847/434-8000
Website: http://www.aap.org

The American Academy of Pediatrics is an organization of pediatricians committed to the attainment of optimal physical, mental, and social health and well-being for all infants, children, adolescents, and young adults. This site is not specifically devoted to children's pain issues, but the keyword "Pain" will access a broad spectrum of information.

## PAIN MEDICATIONS

**MedicineNet.com**
Website: http://www.medicinenet.com

**Medline Plus**
Website: http://www.nlm.hih.gov/medlineplus/druginfo/uspdi/202319.html

# Index

sympathetic nervous system and, 46

therapeutic exercise and, 50

transcutaneous electrical nerve stimulation (TENS) and, 50

nonsteroidal anti–inflammatory drugs (NSAIDs), 55, 58–61, 113, 116

Norco. *See* hydrocodone

norepinephrine, **34**, 40, **41**

Norgesic, 59*t*

Norpramin. *See* desipramine

nortriptyline (Pamelor), 87, 88*t*

Nubain. *See* nalbuphine

nucleus gigantocellularis (NG), 37

nucleus raphe magnus (NRM), 37

numeric rating scale (NRS), 11, **11**

Numorphan. *See* oxymorphone

NyQuil, 59*t*

opioid analgesics. 63–82, 71*t*

addiction, tolerance and, 77–82

adverse effects of, 64

agonist and mixed agonist-antagonist group of, 75

allergic reactions to, 66

buprenorphine (Buprenex, Suboxone) as, 72*t*, 75

butorphanol (Stadol) as, 72*t*, 75

ceiling doses for, 81–82

codeine as, 63, 67–68

constipation as adverse effect of, 64–65

dezocine (Dalgan) as, 72*t*, 75

dihydrocodeine (Panlor) as, 63, 68

dosing evaluations for, 70

effectiveness of, limits to, 81–82

fentanyl (Duragesic) as, 73–74, 75

general principles for use of, 67

hydrocodone (Vicodin, Lortab, Norco) as, 63, 68

hydromorphone (Dilaudid) as, 73, 75

legal ramifications of use of, 63–64

levorphanol as, 72*t*

lifespan and, 80–81

meperidine (Demerol) as, 74–75

methadone (Dolophine) as, 70, 75

morphine as, 63, 69–70, 75

myths concerning use of, 77–82

nalbuphine (Nubain) as, 72*t*, 75

oxycodone (Percocet, Percodan) as, 73

pentazocine (Talwin) as, 72*t*, 75

propoxyphene (Darvon, Darvocet) as, 63, 68

recreational use of, 66

side effects of, 65–66

toxicity of, 66

tramadol (Ultram, Ultracet) as, 69

underutilization of, 63–64, 77–82

oral agents, 57–61, 95–96

Oramorph. *See* morphine

Orudis, 59*t*

oxcarbazepine (Trileptal), 85

oxycodone (Percocet, Percodan), 71*t*, 73

OxyContin. *See* oxycodone

oxymorphone as, 71*t*

pain

acute, 2–3, 15, 54

allodynia and, 6

central nervous system (CNS) and, 4, 26–44, 26

central pattern of distribution of, 4

chronic, 3, 14–15, 54

classification or types of, 2–7

definition of, 1–7

depression, psychological issues, and, 6–7, 20, 23–24

duration, frequency, and pattern of, 14–16, **15**

factitious, or malingering, 7

focal, 3

hormonal fluctuations and, 119

idiopathic, 7

intensity (level) of, 10–12, 54–55

location and distribution of, 13–14, **13**

multifocal, 3

nerve, nerve roots and, 4, 26–27, **27**, 32, 40–44, **42**

neuropathic, 6

nociceptive, 5–6, 38–40, **39**

perception of, individual characteristics and, 1–2

peripheral components of normal pain pathway in, 26–31, **32**

persistent or chronic. *See* chronic pain

ctionmber

Index

Vioxx. *See* rofecoxib
visceral pain, 5
visual analogue scale (VAS), 11, **11**

Wellbutrin. *See* bupropion
wind-up phenomenon, 36–37
women and pain management,
    117–120
World Health Organization pain
    management ladder, 55, **55**
Wygesic, 59*t*

x-rays, 102
Xylocaine, 56

Zanaflex. *See* tizanidine
Zelnorm, 65*t*
ziconotide (Prialt), 99
Zoloft. *See* sertraline
Zonegran. *See* zonisamide
zonisamide (Zonegran), 85
Zostrix. *See* capsaicin
Zydone, 59*t*